INTIMACY, CHANGE,
AND OTHER THERAPEUTIC MYSTERIES

Intimacy, Change, and Other Therapeutic Mysteries

Stories of Clinicians and Clients

David C. Treadway

The Guilford Press

New York   London

Printed in the United States of America

This book is printed on acid-free paper.

Last digit is print number: 9   8   7   6   5   4   3   2   1

Library of Congress Cataloging-in-Publication Data

Treadway, David C.
  Intimacy, change, and other therapeutic mysteries : stories of clinicians and
clients / David C. Treadway.
       p. cm.
  Includes bibliographical references.
  ISBN 1-59385-074-3 (hardcover : alk. paper)
  1. Psychotherapy—Case studies.   2. Psychotherapy patients—Case studies.
I. Title.
  RC465.T74 2004
  616.89′14—dc22

                                                                                    2004013205

ABOUT THE AUTHOR

David C. Treadway, PhD, is a nationally known workshop leader, Director of the Treadway Training Institute, and the author of *Before It's Too Late: Working with Substance Abuse in the Family* and *Dead Reckoning: A Therapist Confronts His Own Grief*. An award-winning contributor to the *Psychotherapy Networker* and other journals, he has appeared on *20/20, Good Morning America*, and other national television programs, and has hosted a radio show on family issues for PBS. Dr. Treadway is in private practice in Weston, Massachusetts (*www.drdavidtreadway.com*), and currently specializes in couple therapy and workshops that support therapists in their own journeys, both personal and professional. He has been happily married for 37 years to Dr. Kate Treadway and is the proud father of two sons, Michael and Sam.

PREFACE

Yesterday was a brute of a day. I felt tired and good. Despite having had to organize an emergency hospitalization in between sessions, I was focused and fully present in each hour. I've been practicing for 30 years. I felt like an old pro.

Then, just as I was about to shut off my office light, the call came from Billy McIntyre.

Five years ago I met with the McIntyre family after the father had killed himself just before his daughter's wedding. The daughter, Heather, had broken off her engagement because she was so shattered. The family and I had a few meetings, and then Heather and I worked together for a year. She was able to do some deep grieving work. I felt very connected to her, partially as a result of my mother's committing suicide when I was about Heather's age. Our work ended when Heather decided to start her life over again by going to graduate school in California. I had thought she was in great shape.

Last year, I got a letter from a Mrs. Eric Svenson from Los Angeles. Enclosed was a photo of Heather holding a little baby girl. Standing close to her with his arm protectively around her was a giant of a man with a mass of curly blonde hair and a smile as big as California. On the back of the picture she wrote,

Dear Dr. Treadway,

I am so lucky. I couldn't resist sending this to you. Aren't they both perfect! I am so happy. But you know, if it hadn't have been for

Daddy, this never would have happened. It makes me feel guilty sometimes. You're the only one I could tell. I knew you'd understand.

Thanks for everything,

Heather

And I did understand. If her father hadn't killed himself, she would have married the other young man and had an entirely different life. If my mother hadn't precipitously killed herself, I never would have been drawn to this profession, my life's work. Heather's letter made me smile at the serendipity of it all.

The call was from her brother, Billy. He said in a flat monotone, "Mom thought you should know. Heather is in the hospital. She took a serious overdose. Looks like she'll be there for a while. Her doctor said. . . . "

I was stunned. What happened to the smiling couple holding the baby and the spirited, upbeat letter she had written? I thought back over the work I had done with Heather. Two years later, she tries to kill herself. Did I miss something? Was she reaching out in the letter?

I decided to go for a walk. Our usually busy road was deserted. Only the snow crunching under my feet broke the silence. I thought of Heather, lying in a hospital bed. How would things turn out? Thirty years from this moment, Heather might be peacefully rocking her newest grandchild to sleep, this suicide attempt just a distant memory. Or she might just as easily end up rocking back and forth in the back ward of a mental hospital.

I didn't feel like an old pro anymore, just old.

Looking up at the black sky, I saw the rising moon. It was not quite full, which gave the man up there a somewhat lopsided head. There was a slight smile playing over his ghostly white face, as if he knew a lot more than I ever would. I felt suddenly very small and insignificant. Oddly enough, it was a comfort. After all, I was just a bit player in Heather's story. For the many harsh and unexpected outcomes I'd seen in my career, there had been just as many miracles. I reminded myself how little we actually know about the people we treat and the results of what we do. Appreciating the enigma of therapy lies in understanding that therapy itself can be powerful, both positively and negatively, even though we who practice it are not. There are always more questions than answers.

I wrote this collection of short stories for clinicians of all kinds. I use these stories to explore the complexity of people's lives, ours as well as our clients', to delve into the often inexplicable impact therapy has on clients and the effect being a therapist has on our own lives. What is the connection between what we think is going on and the experience of the other participants in the room? What happens outside the sessions to clients and therapists alike? How much do our own life experiences determine our response to any given situation, and how does our clinical work affect our personal lives? How do we understand the impact of therapy over time?

When I became a family therapist, I believed passionately in what I did and was arrogant enough to presume that there was a right way and a wrong way to treat families. That seems like a long time ago. In the past 25 years we have reexamined families and therapy from the feminist, deconstructionist, narrative, and biological perspectives, and we have begun to recognize how limited our understanding is about the nature of therapy. We know our clinical calling is more a work of art and an act of love than the practice of science. Our dilemma is that we don't know hour by hour, case by case, which are the constructive sessions that make a real difference. How many of us have felt we have had great sessions, only to have the client drop out of treatment? Conversely, we've all had a session that blew up in our faces only to discover later that that particular session was the turning point for the family. After 30 years of practice, I feel humbled by the mystery of therapy itself.

Years ago I conducted a little research project to assess the correlations among the therapist's perception of the therapy, the clients' perceptions, and the observable results of therapy. A trained family therapist interviewed many of my former clients and recorded their notions about what happened in the therapy. She also observed these clients with her trained eye and made her own independent assessment of how well they were doing. Then she interviewed me without telling me the families' experiences and recorded my recollections of the cases.

The results were startling. Here's a brief summary of some of the responses.

The mother in one family reported, "Dr. Treadway saved our lives. We would never have made it without him." The two adult children and the father nodded in solemn agreement. Yet my researcher observed that the daughter was still anorectic, the son belligerent and living at home at 25, the father reeked of alcohol, and the mother was frantically trying to manage everyone. My recollection was that the therapy ended with no progress because the family's insurance ran out.

Another family that I considered one of my stellar success stories reported that the therapy had been ineffectual but their situation had dramatically improved during the same time period because they had started attending church regularly together.

The *coup de grâce* was the interview with my former client, Susan Murray. I had fond memories of my 18 sessions with Sue, who came at the behest of her parents her first week of freshman year at Wellesley. I don't have daughters, and I liked Sue immensely. I remember trying to be a wise, kindly, safe man, *in loco parentis*, who might help her navigate a way through the treacherous waters of her first year of college.

Sue was in law school when she said the following to my researcher: "Oh, I remember Dr. Treadwell. He was a shrink my parents made me see a couple of times during the first few weeks of college. I don't actually remember whether or not it was helpful. He was a nice enough man, though." Then she paused before saying, "Oh, wait, I do remember something. One night he walked me to my car because it was late and the parking lot light wasn't on. I remember he said something incredible. At the time, I felt like it changed my life."

My researcher asked, "What did he say?"

"Oh, gee, I don't remember."

And when my interviewer asked me, I didn't even remember the walk to the car.

Did that one therapeutic moment really change Sue's life? What role does therapy play in helping people change their lives, anyway? Did my work with Heather truly help her? Is it hubris to think that what we do makes any difference at all?

Obviously life itself is a steady stream of change as we go through the normal developmental stages. Yet sometimes change can be sudden and discontinuous, often precipitated by a traumatic event like a near-death experience, loss of a loved one, or a family crisis. Usually people enter therapy when they are experiencing some kind of crisis and are in pain. Pain is nature's warning signal that something is wrong and needs to be addressed. And yet it is often unclear whether our clients need the pain ameliorated or utilized as a prompt to make significant changes in their lives.

If a client is depressed because she's trapped in a marriage with a high-functioning alcoholic and she's trying to raise three young children, how do we judge what's most helpful? How do we decide which approach is better and for whom? Suppose we challenge the wife to confront the husband in the hopes of precipitating his recovery. Maybe he gets sober or maybe the wife is impelled toward a divorce. Who is better off: the alcoholic, the wife, the kids? I once helped a family practice "tough love" with one of its members whom they had been forcing in and out of alcohol treatment ineffectively for years. I encouraged them to let go and let him take responsibility for his own recovery, the standard intervention of the time. The family did it. But he didn't commit himself into treatment; he broke off his relationships with the family and drank himself to death.

It's almost impossible to judge the impact of what we do and how it influences people's choices in the long run. My wife and I have been together for 37 years, but if we hadn't been so codependent and enmeshed when we married in our early 20s the couple therapy we did back then probably would have led us to splitting up. Instead we left the therapy and stayed together. This leaves us oddly grateful now for our interwoven neuroses that were as much the glue that held us together as true love. On the other hand, I was instrumental in holding together a marriage that now, 15 years later, both spouses have said to me they wished they had ended. In our last session, when these two people, now in their late sixties, were acknowledging to each other that they felt it had been a mistake to stay together, we all wept.

In addition to exploring the complexity and confusion of our work with our clients, these stories help us consider the effect our own lives have on the therapy we do. Sometimes when my wife and I aren't being particularly intimate I find myself reassuring my couples that relationships can't always be close and it's natural that there can be sexual dry spells. So who is reassuring whom? We need to consider how our life experience, gender, and personal beliefs affect our treatment. If we have divorced successfully, are we prone to encourage that as an option? If we have stuck out a difficult marriage, do we sell the value of commitment? I believe we are all prone to promoting our own solutions, either consciously or unconsciously. There is no way to predict accurately when our particular subjectivity is helpful or harmful to the people we treat.

This book asks us how being a therapist affects the unfolding of our own lives. My colleague Mike Elkin used to say, "Therapists are the only people who seem to need thirty or more hours of therapy a week."

In the eyes of the public, we are perceived either as paragons of virtue or crazier than our patients. Who are we really, and how does our work shape our lives and our relationships?

In some respects, the therapeutic role allows many of us to experience a tremendous degree of daily intimacy. From the safety of the therapist's chair, we can risk loving our clients and engaging them at the most vulnerable level of their lives. Having come from a family shattered by suicide, mental illness, and addiction, I am painfully aware that being a therapist provided a safe venue for me to do my own healing. I found safety and comfort in helping my clients work through their grief. I borrowed their tears until I was strong enough to shed my own.

It's also true that it's easier to be intimate in therapy than it sometimes is in our own relationships as partners and parents. At times throughout my career I have realized that I have given my best love in the office and have precious little left over for my wife, children, and friends. On one side of my home office door I can be patient, tender, and kind, and yet on the other side of the door, if one of my kids fiddled with his food at dinner, I might have snapped his head off. What is the cost to those we're closest to, when we give our all at the office? I remember all the times I glanced out the window past my clients and saw my older son when he was little, sitting by himself on the swing set. Now, he's 24 and gone. My clients are still in my office. The swings are empty.

Therapy is a temporary, intermittent engagement between flawed and struggling human beings immersed in the complexity of their own lives. No wonder it is virtually impossible to figure out its impact.

I began to write this book because in the heart of every clinical hour is a unique story. I wanted to capture the ineffable mystery of people and of the powerful and unexpected consequences of therapy. The power of the short stories is that they allow us to look at the prism of people's lives. As novelist Tim O'Brien says, "Writing fiction involves a desire to enter the mystery of things, the human craving to know what cannot be known."

Intimacy, Change, and Other Therapeutic Mysteries is not a book of case studies. Nor is it a book of research that reports the clients' experience. Too often our diagnostic codes, research studies, and case presentations risk reducing people's stories down to a formula. They also tend to reinforce the us/them split between therapist and clients. This a book of stories in which the lives of clients and therapists are seen unfolding side by side. We not only see what is happening between people, but we can also enter the complex internal experiences of all the participants. Often we see the same moment from the differing perspectives of the therapists and the clients, each with his or her own subjective truths.

The stories take us beyond the therapy room to how the therapy affects both clinicians and clients in their lives outside the session. Some of the stories revisit the lives of characters from earlier stories, illuminating the myriad ways people change over time. Other stories are only peripherally about therapy and describe moments and circumstances that are turning points in people's lives.

These stories are fiction inspired by my work but not based on particular cases. They also don't reflect a broad range of clinical issues or a very diverse population. Many of the stories revolve around issues of intimacy and grief that affect clinicians and clients alike. In creating these stories that aspire to show the courage and character, suffering and love that are a part of all of our lives, I hope I have honored those whom I have been privileged to know.

I wrote this book for both graduate students and seasoned therapists. No matter how sophisticated and experienced we might be, the fundamental questions about the work we do still need to be raised. Any given case can make us feel like raw beginners again. Continually questioning what we do is a way of seeing ourselves and our clients with the awe and openness that Zen teachers refer to as "beginner's mind."

At the end of the book there is a Study Guide that shows how the stories could be used in seminars, peer supervision, and book groups. I offer questions at the end of each story to provoke thought and discussion, not just about the story but also about our own clients and feelings about ourselves as therapists. I hope the questions will challenge the readers to find their own truth about the work they do. Also at the end of the book, there is a section of Suggested Readings that lists several references about the topics raised in each story.

One of my colleagues challenged me about writing a book that generates only questions. "These questions are great, but you're a very senior-level therapist; certainly you've got some of your own answers about this stuff. Why aren't you putting them in there?"

Over the years, I haven't been fully satisfied with my own answers. But I can't ask the readers to address these issues if I am unwilling to risk exposing my own thoughts. All of us have to have a set of values and beliefs about who we are and the profession we practice. We have to take responsibility for both the good and the harm that we might do. At the end of the book, I reflect on how I have struggled with these issues throughout my clinical life and offer my own ideas about the complexity of our work and how it affects us as well as our clients. I don't offer answers, just one man's opinions after a lifetime of practice.

I get up to refill my coffee mug. It's time to prepare for my session. I don't usually see Saturday clients but I had to fit one case in this morning. I used to see Heather on Saturdays because it was the only time she had available. Thoughts of her keep popping into my mind. I didn't expect to be writing about her.

The couple I'm about to see upsets me. They've got three young kids and they're throwing away their marriage just because it doesn't fulfill all their emotional needs. As if any marriage could. Why am I feeling so critical? Am I reacting to Heather and her willingness to throw away her own life? Is some of my old anger at my mother's suicide creeping in?

Soon the couple will be sitting stiffly at either end of my blue sofa like metal book ends. Behind their cold and angry masks, I know there will be such pain and despair in each of their eyes. Where is my compassion?

Outside my window a rosy glow catches my eye. I remember my colleague Nancy's morning meditation. She always starts her day with a prayer: "Please, God, let me see the people who will sit before me today through Your eyes."

I pause. I think of Heather and all the other people whose lives I have been fortunate to be a part of for a while. I think of all of us who practice this arcane art. What happens in therapy may be a mystery. But therapists aren't. We are people with a calling: people who risk opening our hearts to the suffering of others. We believe that being one caring person, in one session, even one moment can sometimes be the difference that makes a difference.

I think again of the lost and hurting couple I'll see in the next few minutes. I bow my head and whisper Nancy's prayer.

ACKNOWLEDGMENTS

Perhaps it does take a village to raise an author. Needless to say, saying thank you seems a barely adequate response to the many people who have made this book possible. Jim Nageotte, my editor at The Guilford Press, has been a believer in this project from the beginning. Jim, thank you for your encouragement, guidance, and enthusiasm.

Cindy Barrilleaux, a writing coach and associate editor of *Psychotherapy Networker*, was the midwife for the project. She was with me over every single line written. Truly she was my coauthor and partner. No one could have critiqued my work with such inspiration, acumen, and kindness. Cindy, you helped me face my limitations and bring out the best that I could do. And we had fun all the way through. Thanks also to my many other writing coaches and supporters, particularly Leslie Lawrence and the group, Dennis Palumbo, Rich Simon, Barry Dym, and Jay Lappin.

Special thanks to my therapist, Nancy Riemer, who has been as steady as a heartbeat throughout this effort. Nancy, our work has sustained me in this work. I wouldn't have been able to do this book without our therapy.

To my 91-year-old father, who has been steadfast in his support of this project, I want to say, "Even an old guy like me needs fatherly guidance and encouragement. Thanks, Dad, for being there."

My two sons, Michael and Sam, have also been there for me, as writing this book has absorbed my time like a sponge. Each of them has conveyed understanding and appreciation for the endeavor while putting up their sometimes irascible old man.

Last, I give special thanks to my wife, Dr. Kate Treadway, who has been a gift to me throughout my adult life. The present of her presence has made my life possible. Thank you, Kate, for everything. And I mean every thing.

CONTENTS

1988

1988

LUNAR MISSIONS

I

"God, I hope he doesn't bring home flowers," Kim thought as she glanced over at Sarah working on her science project. She was hoping that Bob wouldn't try anything just because it was the night before a therapy session. It would be hard to say no. She knew she'd be in trouble if he came in and gave her a big hug and a bouquet of red roses. He always tried the roses, even when they were out of season. They used to be her favorite.

Kim shuddered at the anticipation of Bob's overture. Sometimes his amorous attention reminded her of her dad when he was in the cuddles phase of his drinking. He would slobber affection on her. He even did it when she was a teenager, and in front of her best friends, too. Like when he barged into her room when they were playing with her Tarot cards on her bed, yanked her up, and gave her a big squeeze, "How's my little girl today?" while Kara and Susie kept their eyes glued on their cards.

"Mom! Mom! Get Daddy out of here."

Her mom's shadow appeared at the door with a whisper, "Now, Ted, girls don't like being hugged, especially in front of their friends. Come along."

She wished she could hide under her bed like she did when she was little. Holding her breath.

Mom pulled him out of there and we heard them arguing their way down the hall. "I wasn't doing anything wrong. I was just giving her some cuddles. We could use a little more affection around this house."

"Shhh, Ted."

Kim grimaced at the memory of her father's ruddy face, the reek of the stale blend of sweat, cigarettes, and whiskey, and watching her friends stare at him out of the corner of their eyes. Then she shook her head. It wasn't as if Bob was asking her to fly to the moon. If he was up for it, she could do it too. Maybe it will show they were making progress.

"Was it Armstrong or Aldrin who took the first step, Mom?"

"I'm not sure, sweetie, but I think it was Armstrong," Kim replied, looking over at her earnest daughter at the breakfast table, surrounded by a pile of reference books. It was Sarah's first big research project and she wouldn't be happy just getting the details right. She wanted her report on the Apollo project to be the best in her class. Kim was so proud of her and couldn't help wishing that a little of his sister's academic discipline would rub off on Bobby, who was sitting in front of the tube watching "The Brady Bunch."

Kim's husband, Bob Dunbar, was stuck in traffic in the light rain. Creeping along in the passing lane always agitated Bob, but more than the traffic irritated him today. He was mad at himself for flirting with his new young secretary again. Maria was pretty and sweet and all together too willing. Like this morning, when she brought him his coffee: She must have known he was looking down the front of her low-cut blouse as she bent over to place the cup on his desk. And maybe she could even tell that the scent of her freshly shampooed hair spilling forward toward him made him think of her naked in the shower.

"Well, Miss Riggoti, nobody makes a better cup of coffee. You have the magic touch."

"So does that mean that I've earned the right to be called Maria, Mr. Dunbar?" she questioned teasingly.

"Only when you'll start calling me Bob."

"Mr. Dunbar, I couldn't do that. After all," she said, and lowered her voice to a throaty whisper, "you're my boss."

The honking startled Bob and he glanced up to see the green light. In his rearview mirror there was a silver Porsche Carrera with an annoyed bald man waving him on impatiently. He couldn't believe he was toying with such a classic midlife cliché as chasing after his secretary. Worst of all, he wasn't at all sure that he could handle it if they did start something. Christ, he'd be better off buying the Porsche. He knew he could handle a car.

He had never cheated on Kim, but in the last few years, since their sex life had evaporated, it had become harder and harder for Bob to stay faithful. It really wasn't either the sex or the person that tugged at him so hard. It was the thrill of being desired. Kim didn't want him at all anymore, and probably took his fidelity for granted no matter how sporadic their lovemaking. Bob guessed that his loyalty was motivated as much by fear as honor. He couldn't bear the thought of losing Kim. The possibility that the couple therapy with Dr. Evans might be the beginning of the end had already crossed his mind.

The therapy was Kim's idea. Bob wanted to rekindle their sex life, but it wasn't clear how talking about it was going to help. It made him even more self-conscious. He particularly didn't like the therapeutic exercises where they were supposed to take turns telling each other what they would like to change in their sex life. They hadn't done it yet and the session was the next day. What was he supposed to say to her? "Gee, Kim, seems like sex is one of your least favorite household chores, like folding laundry or polishing the brass." How is saying stuff like that going to help? Besides, after that night three years ago, there had been virtually no sex at all.

Remembering what happened made Bob shudder: the sight of the shock and horror in her eyes when she walked in on him. They had never talked about it. He knew he wouldn't bring it up. But clearly it had an impact on their sex life. Kim simply lost all interest after that fiasco.

Maybe we can do something tonight, he thought. I know she

doesn't want to look bad in front of Evans. And besides, it's been weeks.

He glanced at the snazzy array of pansies sitting in the front seat next to him. A surprise. He had certainly never brought these home before.

Unlike Bob Dunbar's, Dr. Jack Evans's commute was just a few steps from his office to the kitchen. Jack closed the door on the noisy mess of a family he had just wrestled with for an hour and pumped his fist. Days end!

Then there was a tentative knock. "Just a minute, Alex," he called out to his six-year-old daughter. He walked back to the clutter on his desk and looked at his next day's lineup as he always did. Bob and Kim Dunbar were first up. Good couple, Jack thought before he swung the door wide open. Alex bounced into the room. "I've done all my homework. Can we work on our puzzle now?"

Jack sighed. Sometimes he wished he had a short commute so he had a little time to switch gears.

"Please, Daddy, pretty please." She smiled up at him. She was always at her best when her big sister wasn't around.

Jack put her down, glanced back at the list of unanswered phone calls and said, "Sure, sweetie, maybe we can finally find the rest of the edge pieces tonight."

II

Bob was stretched out on their bed and flipping through *Time* magazine while he waited for Kim to get out of the bath. It was always a good sign when she took a bath. But sometimes she spent so long, it was like she was hiding out in there.

He remembered guiltily stealing a peek at his mother in the bath through a crack in the door. She had her eyes closed and she seemed so peaceful. He studied every detail of her naked body, the black patch of hair between her legs and particularly her breasts with the raised dark nipples that protruded out of the water like islands. He was just 11 and the exciting tingle in his erection was still surprising.

A month later when his father told him she had advanced breast cancer and would have a double mastectomy, shame flushed his face red and he ran out of the room. Probably his dad just thought he was upset with the news, but his first response was a spasm of shame about how he had stared at her.

No one talked about her illness. She lost her hair and wore a wig. She lost weight. She was nauseous all the time. But she just acted like the mom she always used to be: helping him with school projects and still baking him treats she called "Bobby Surprises."

Once that last spring, she was sitting out on the porch swing. He came out and she was looking really tired and thin. She didn't look like his mom at all. She saw him standing by the door. "Come out here, Bobby. Sit with me for a bit." He sat down next to her and she put an arm around him. She was in an old black tank top that just drooped off her, and her arm seemed as light as a bird's wing. She didn't say anything. They just swung there for a while and then he said, "I've got to go do my homework."

"It's okay, Bobby, I want you to always do well in school," and she gave him a weak little squeeze.

After she died, Bob's older brother and father were very stoical, but Bob was devastated. He had been dumb enough to believe she was going to get better. He moped around the house, and at bedtime, no matter how hard he tried not to, he cried into his pillow.

"Shut up, sissy," his brother grumbled from the lower bunk. "Crying isn't going to bring her back."

Bob used to sneak into his parents' bedroom just to stand in her closet. She had rows of dresses, suits, and skirts in there, and he could remember her in most of them, particularly the black velvet dress she always wore on Christmas Eve. On one side of the door she had a shoe rack filled with high heels, flats, and her jogging sneakers. On the other side hung her nightgown and her bed jacket. He stood there inhaling the pungent blend of shoe leather and old perfume. It smelled like her. Sometimes he opened her bureau and looked through her lingerie, jewelry, blouses, and sweaters. It was strangely comforting to touch her things. Once he picked up a pair of her nylon tricot panties and gently caressed his cheek with them. They were so soft. Suddenly he took off his pants and underwear and pulled the panties on. Touching himself through the silky material gave him a shuddering thrill and the shock of his first orgasm. It felt so good that he did it again despite feeling very ashamed. For a while, he actually hid a pair of her panties in the back of his sock drawer. After the intense stimulation, the moment would always end in a rush of sadness and he would just plain miss her. In the end, the nauseous dread of being discovered stopped him. He imagined how it would feel if his brother or father caught him in the act.

Kim was the first girl to touch him. He had always been so frightened of girls that he never even kissed anyone in high school. Kim seemed so experienced. And she was a sophomore when he was a freshman at Middlebury.

In the back seat of her father's Impala, she guided his hands to her breasts and gently taught him how to caress. When she reached down to his crotch, he came immediately. "It's okay," she whispered, "I know about boys being quick. We'll practice."

And they did, everywhere and anywhere. But sometimes she was almost too much for him to handle.

One Saturday, they had her house to themselves and they spent the day in her bedroom with posters of Jimi Hendrix, Jim Morrison, and Mick Jagger staring at them. The third time they did it she had insisted on being on top of him and he felt almost smothered. Her breasts loomed over him as she ground into his pelvis. She grimaced as she worked for her orgasm.

Afterwards he asked, "Do you always like to do it this much?"

"What are you saying?" she exclaimed. Then she turned her back to him and was quiet.

"I, ah, am sorry, ah. . . . "

"Never mind. It's nothing. I'm just tired. I need a nap before my parents get home."

That was the last time they ever did it more than once at a time.

Kim lay in the bath and examined her body. "I'm just too fat," she thought. She cupped her breasts in her hands and looked at each one in turn. They'd never been the same after Bobby nursed them to death. She used to be proud of them. And she knew that Bob got a big kick out of them. When they were first dating, she would wear a push-up bra under a low-cut silk blouse and he would go nuts over her. She smiled at the thought. But now her breasts were clearly at the mercy of gravity and time. There were even sag lines, as if her skin was getting tired of holding them up.

Kim let herself settle down into the soothing softness and lilac smell of her bubble bath. She knew Bob was waiting. He was probably lying there on the bed without any clothes. Seeing him in the nude sometimes reminded her of that time with her father. She woke up with a jolt when he flicked on her bedroom light and there he was dead drunk, swaying back and forth, and naked all over. He collapsed on her bed and passed out. Kim turned her back to him and pretended to be asleep. She stayed awake watching the luminous hands on the clock slowly circle toward morning.

When her father sat down to breakfast, she studied his face, waiting to see if he'd show her a sign about what happened. Nothing. Except he didn't even give a glance her way. He munched through his Wheaties and stuck his head into the sports pages. Her mother bustled about like a worker bee on speed. No one said anything about anything at all.

Kim sighed. Bob was probably getting impatient, but she just wasn't ready. Yet. She needed a little more time.

Bob was impatient waiting for Kim to finish her bath. He felt the early stirrings of arousal in his groin. He was thinking about Maria and the flash of her shimmering thighs when she crossed her legs. He wished he was thinking that way about Kim.

The last session with Evans disturbed Bob.

"Now this may seem a little strange, but I'd like you to turn to each other and share a particularly favorite memory of when you felt both intimate and sexual with each other," Evans said in his friendly, "aw-shucks" style.

"Well, I remember the time Bob told me about how close he was to his mother before she got sick and he began to cry, which he never does. I felt really close to him and I held him and then the next thing you know we were, you know."

Evans smiled and turned to Bob and said, "So, do you remember that special time?"

Bob sensed that Evans was looking to create some kind of emotional reconnection between them right then and there. But his feelings about that moment were quite different. He'd been embarrassed about bawling like a baby, and completely taken aback when Kim began to touch him in a sexual way. He remembered wanting to jump out of the bed, but he submitted because she was being so loving and he didn't want to hurt her feelings.

"Oh sure," he said as he turned away from Kim and responded to Evans. "It was nice even though I had been embarrassed about crying."

Thankfully, Evans let him off the hook. Even Kim seemed to get that they were in deep water. But he could tell that Evans had noticed his discomfort. Later in the session, Evans said something about wanting to know more about his relationship with his mother.

Kim avoided looking at herself in the mirror as she toweled off. She was trying to remember where she had last seen her diaphragm. That's right, she thought, it's in my overnight bag from our anniversary outing. What a disaster. The romantic country inn with a fireplace in the room and a canopied double bed, and all they did was have a miserable fight.

Putting in the diaphragm always irritated Kim. She couldn't imagine anything less romantic than putting her leg on the toilet, greasing the cup, then shoving it up there. It seemed so mechanical. Like sex with Bob. Now, it was mostly just going through the motions.

In the beginning it had been fine. He was so inexperienced that she had fun playing the sophisticated older woman. Bob was the first boy with whom she had felt comfortable being intimate. He hadn't pawed at her the way the others did, and she enjoyed feeling in charge.

But she vaguely remembered that he seemed to get more uptight as time went by. After a while he'd always turn her down if she initiated, yet he expected her to respond when he was in the mood. It felt like he just wanted to have sex for the release and it didn't have anything to do with her. His approach was kind of apologetic and whiney, and he always managed to remind her about how long it had been since their last time.

Then, a few years ago, she had come home early from work and surprised Bob in their bedroom. She came around the corner and there he was, standing in front of their mirror dressed in her bra, panties, stockings, and her favorite chemise. He looked like a frantic trapped animal.

"What are you doing?" she blurted out in horror.

But he ran into the bathroom and slammed the door. The sight of his mad dash to the bathroom in her lingerie made him look even more pathetic and ridiculous. She felt like throwing open the door and screaming, but she knew she couldn't stand seeing him again that way so she turned on her heels and marched out of the room.

Later he came down for family dinner and they acted like nothing happened. They'd never spoken of it since. She tried to put it out of her mind, but she often found herself remembering him and the desperate look on his face every time she wore that particular chemise. The image of him in her underclothes mostly disgusted her, but sometimes she found herself feeling sorry for him. He must have been so mortified. So ashamed. She'd catch herself looking at him as his regular self—driving, doing the dishes, or helping the kids with their homework—and wonder, what was it all about? What possible charge could he get from putting on her underwear? Was he really one of those transvestites you see on the "Phil Donahue" show? And what does he think about what happened? She was actually relieved that he never brought it up. And she wasn't about to broach it. Finally she just threw the stupid chemise out.

She wondered if the episode would come up in the therapy. She was sure Bob wasn't going to mention it. What would Dr. Evans think? On the other hand, maybe we better let that sleeping dog lie, she thought.

Kim pushed the harsh memories out of her mind and began debating whether to wear the lacy black negligee that Bob gave her for

Christmas. She remembered that when she opened it she wondered irritably, is this item for me or for him? She hardly ever wore it, but decided tonight was the night. Bob would be so pleased.

For a moment, she imagined him reporting to Dr. Evans that things were actually getting better after all. Maybe Evans could help him really open up.

Kim felt okay about Evans so far. He had picked up on Bob's discomfort and was working hard to make a connection with him. He seemed quite empathic about the sexual pressures she felt. Pretty tuned in for a man. Kim would have preferred to work with a woman therapist, but she couldn't imagine Bob going to a woman. Therapy was hard enough for him.

She opened the bathroom door and stood on the threshold for a moment, waiting to catch Bob's eye. He didn't look up from his magazine. She felt a familiar tension in her chest.

When Bob saw her come toward him in the negligee, he reached over to pull back the covers on her side of the bed and smiled. "I thought maybe you drowned in there," he said.

"I wasn't in there that long."

"I know, honey. I'm just fooling around. The suspense was killing me."

"What suspense?"

"You know, I wasn't sure whether we were going to do anything tonight or not."

"What makes you think that we are?" Kim teased.

"Aren't we? I mean, I thought the nightgown, you know, meant that. . . . "

"It's all right, don't panic." Kim slipped into bed. She turned toward him and gave him a smile. He scooted over, put his arms around her, and leaned toward her for a kiss.

"Hold on a second," Kim stopped him. "You know we haven't done our therapy assignment about talking with each other."

"For god sake, we're not going to do that now."

"Well, okay, but it's not my fault. I brought it up three times," Kim said quickly. "By the way, did you get the cat in?"

"Of course, I got the cat in."

"And did you say goodnight to Sarah and Bobby? I don't want them wandering in here."

"Kim, I said goodnight and told them we were going to sleep, okay? What else do you want me to do, put on the burglar alarm?"

Kim patted his cheek and said, "Don't get mad, I'm just trying to switch gears."

"Well, your love talk doesn't exactly drive me wild."

"Let's not talk anymore," she whispered. She moved closer and put her hands between his legs. She felt his flaccid penis and said, "Gee, you're not exactly a raging bull yourself."

"What do you expect? It's not a big turn-on to go over your nightly list of chores."

"I give up!" Kim turned her back to him. "I just can't do this."

"Hey, come on, I'm sorry, I'm a little nervous. Let's keep trying," Bob said as gently as he could.

Kim lay curled up with her back to him in silence. She wished she had put on her flannel nightgown and skipped the whole idea. She felt as silly as a Barbie doll in her frilly negligee.

Part of Bob wanted to just roll over and forget about it too, but opportunities to have sex had been so few and far between that he was loath to let go of this one, even though he wasn't the slightest bit turned on. If they didn't try, he'd be even more pissed in the morning.

Very tentatively, he began to massage her back. After a while, he inched his hand around to her breast. Kim shifted her arm slightly to make it easier for him to reach her nipple. It hardened under the touch of his fingers. When she was close enough to being ready, she rolled over and pulled him on top of her. In the dark and silent room, they each retreated to their private fantasies while their bodies pushed against each other. He was too quick.

"I'm sorry," said Bob, breaking the silence. "Do you want me to do you?"

"That's okay, don't worry," Kim said. "At least we did something."

"Well, goodnight then," Bob said, self-consciously yawning and rolling away from her.

13

Kim didn't reply. She lay on her side and pulled her legs up toward her breasts. She decided to not even bother to go to the bathroom. Her mind downshifted toward sleep. She reminded herself to pick up the Con-Tact paper for Sarah's project. Suddenly the image of the first moon landing popped into her head. She could see Neil Armstrong, encased in the bulky white suit, stepping down onto the dusty lunar surface from the landing module. She remembered being curled up in Bob's arms as they watched the black and white images and heard Armstrong say, "That's one small step for man, one giant leap for mankind."

Kim listened to Bob's rhythmic breathing behind her and thought of their therapy session the next morning. Despite her lack of fulfillment, she was glad they'd pulled it off. Mission accomplished, she thought as she drifted off.

III

Ellen Evans brought some coffee up for both of them. She walked into their dressing room and said to Jack, "What are you dressed up for? Are you doing a workshop today?"

"Yup, my regular one: 'Intimacy, Sexuality, and Grief.' You should come sometime. I'll give you a few pointers," he said, turning toward her and reaching for the coffee cup.

"Wow, wisdom from the great Dr. Evans himself. I'd be honored. Although, frankly, my dear," Ellen said tartly, "I'd be happier if you'd just practice a little of what you preach."

Jack looked at her in her bathrobe, with her bed hair spilling all over and the slightly quarrelsome look on her still tired-looking face.

She looked halfway between concern and combat. He always had to remind himself what their therapist, Beth Harney, had told him, to look for the hurt right underneath Ellen's anger.

"Hey, sweetie, I know, guilty as charged. I don't know why I haven't been with the program lately. It's so lame to use the 'I'm too tired approach,' but it's true. I don't know what's going on," he said as he opened his arms to her.

Ellen's face softened and she met his embrace. "I know you're feeling bad, but I don't know what to do," she said.

"Well, unfortunately, I think maybe I should go in and see Dr. Beth. I'm feeling really shut down. You know, after I spend the hours with my clients, I don't feel like I've got anything left over for us."

Ellen stiffened and then pulled away from Jack. "Is there a reason why you want to see her on your own that your not telling me?" she asked.

"Ellen, don't go there, that stuff was a long time ago. You don't have anything to worry about."

"Really?"

"You've got to trust me on this. I would never do that to you again. Ever." Jack opened his arms.

Ellen came to him. "You know I still get scared."

"I know. Maybe we should go back to see Beth together. I really don't have anything to hide."

They hugged.

Ellen left early to beat the commute, and Jack took Megan and Alex to their favorite restaurant for breakfast. While they waited, Alex talked her big sister into another game of Paper, Rock, Scissors.

Alex won and crowed triumphantly, "You're bigger but I'm better."

Jack kept his mouth shut. Telling Alex to stop being mean to her big sister never worked. Just made her worse. Mostly Megan brushed her off as if she were just an annoying housefly. But it bothered Jack that his youngest was so competitive and tough. So much for their special time together. Maybe he should have just put them on the bus.

"You and Ellen overindulge those kids because you're so damn guilty that you both work so hard," lectured his dad, Skipper. "Nobody brought me up. Back in my day, kids raised themselves."

Jack usually cringed when Skipper launched into his parenting tips. Maybe the old man had a point.

Jack sat at his desk going over the lineup for the day. He heard Kim and Bob come into the waiting room and reviewed their file

15

quickly. This was their eighth session. Kim and Bob had moved quickly from the classic "communications" problem to talking about being almost asexual. Jack was worried that things might be moving too quickly. He wasn't sure he'd established the kind of emotional safety net that made it okay for them to deal with intensely vulnerable issues.

As he began to focus on them, he could feel his own bad mood clear like morning fog burned off by the sun. Thank God for clients, he thought, with a rueful smile.

Kim and Bob were a good-looking couple, about the same height, he in his sport jacket and gray flannels and she in one of those red power suits with shoulder pads. He had black wavy hair and a lean, taut face. She had shoulder length blonde hair and deep blue eyes, and her face was completely made up. She had probably dressed up expressly for the session because Jack was sure that she was a stay-at-home mom.

Kim started as soon as they sat down. "Well, we've made some progress, haven't we?" Kim said, and then turned toward Bob expectantly.

"Sure, it's a little better," replied Bob, looking down at the floor.

A shadow of hurt passed across Kim's face. She said brightly, "I'm not suggesting everything is all worked out. All I was saying is that we've made some progress."

Jack felt the tension between them, but was unsure whether it was a good idea to break it wide open so early in the session. He usually began by underlining the positive elements first. "So tell me, both of you, what kind of progress do you feel you have made?"

Kim looked at Bob, but he continued to avoid eye contact with her. She turned back to Jack and said, "Well, we've been avoiding fights. We didn't use that technique of taking turns listening to each other formally, but I feel like we're both listening better. And last night we did manage to do something. At least it was a start."

"So it felt good to fight a little less, and at least you've had one successful encounter in the bedroom," Jack replied, and he turned his swivel chair to face Bob more directly, "And what do you think, Bob?"

"I don't know what I'm supposed to say," he said, as he sat stiffly in his chair. " I feel like you and Kim are waiting for me to be all excited about our encounter last night, when the last time it happened was four months ago and who knows when the next time will be." Then he caught himself, sat up, and said, "I know I shouldn't be so pessimistic. It was good that we tried it. It really was."

"Bob, it's okay for you to keep your guard up and be skeptical. I don't hear Kim suggesting that everything has been fixed," Jack said, searching for a bridge between them. Kim seemed to be shrinking away, looking both hurt and angry. Bob was obviously tense and defensive.

Kim brushed at some lint on her skirt. "Bob doesn't understand that I feel pressure about sex all the time. I mean, he's trying hard not to make a lot of demands, but I know what he wants. Every time we go to bed he goes over to his side of the bed and turns his back to me. I just lie there, looking at his back, and I can tell he's waiting for me to say something or do something. It feels so awful, sometimes I can't even go to sleep until I know he's. . . . "

"What the hell do you expect me to do?" Bob interrupted. "If I ask for it, I'm 'too demanding,' and now you tell me that I'm putting pressure on you even when I don't say anything at all. That's ridiculous!"

"What about last night? Doesn't that mean anything? I'm doing the best I can. I'm just trying to say how it feels. Don't you understand? It makes me feel awful."

"Great, Kim, have your feelings, but what about mine? I suppose I'm not supposed to have any of those either. The only reason why you did it last night was so you could come in here and say you did it."

Bob was glaring at her. Kim began to cry. They both turned and looked at Dr. Evans.

Here we go, Jack thought: They're looking to me for a verdict. I wish Bob could just listen to her for once without getting so defensive. Jack searched for the safe line through these rapids.

"Look, Bob," he said gently, "you have to realize that Kim being upset doesn't mean you're doing anything wrong. You've been trying really hard, too."

Kim and Bob appeared to be settling down. They were both listening intently. Jack turned toward Kim and continued. "And Kim, you need to realize that men often express their hurt feelings by being angry. Let's face it, Bob was taught years ago that only sissies cry, and so even though he hurts on the inside much the same way you do, it just comes out in anger. Unfortunately, men often express too many of their emotional needs through their desire for sex. Bob has the same needs you have to be held, nurtured, and loved. It just gets expressed differently."

The couple sat quietly, reflecting.

This is good, Jack thought as he looked at them both. But they were still radiating plenty of tension.

"You seem to express quite well how men feel, Dr. Evans," Kim said quietly while staring down at the Oriental carpet.

Oh, shit, how did I lose her? Jack thought.

Her lips were pursed tightly. She looked tense and angry. Therapy often felt to Jack like performing the circus act of balancing several spinning plates on sticks at the same time. This plate was falling.

Jack quickly said, "Kim, I'm sorry if it seems like I tune in to Bob better that I do to you. Sometimes I forget you could feel a little ganged up on in here. And I know his needs for sex put a lot of pressure on you."

"Well, I just don't think his 'needs,' as you call them, get expressed so naturally," Kim replied almost in a whisper. "I don't think we would be in such trouble if I hadn't come in on him dressed up in my underwear. . . . "

"Damn it, Kim!" Bob blurted out, "I don't believe you're bringing that up here. For christsake, if you don't shut up I'm walking out. You'd like that, wouldn't you? Then you could blame it all on me. For years you made me feel like shit about sex. Treated me like a beggar. And when you finally agree to do something, you just lay there like a dead animal. But none of that matters. Now you want to tell him it's all me. Well, why don't you just go fuck yourself!"

Silence.

Kim covered her face in her hands and began crying. Bob sat upright on the edge of his seat. He looked like he might bolt out of the room. His face was flushed and his eyes were filled with tears.

Jack almost dropped his notepad, he was so surprised. He couldn't believe the way she dropped this bombshell. It felt as if he moved toward either one of them he'd lose the other.

"Listen, you two, this kind of thing can feel pretty horrible. In a way, it's my fault because we never really talked about what's okay to bring up in therapy," he said, hoping to diffuse some of the intensity. This moment could be a turning point or a disaster and he was afraid of making an irreparable mistake.

"Frankly, Bob, if I were in your shoes, I would really be furious with Kim for exposing you in this way. It makes sense that you would be embarrassed and feel betrayed. And Kim, I know that you didn't mean to humiliate Bob, and that your own hurt and anger just got the better of you," Jack said, hoping it was true.

"I'm sorry, I'm sorry," Kim said, barely audible between sobs.

Bob didn't say anything for a bit. Then he turned to Jack and said quietly, "I don't know if I'm going to come back here. I don't see how this can help anybody."

"You might be right, Bob, but I hope you can hear how bad Kim feels about this. It sounds like this issue has been an impossible thing for you two to talk about or even understand. And clearly this wasn't the way to get into it, but. . . . "

"I knew she was going to do this," Bob interrupted. "You should have seen the look on her face when she came in the room and saw me. She was disgusted. She probably thinks I'm some kind of a pervert. I can't talk about it."

"I didn't know what to think at the time," Kim whispered. "It made my skin crawl. It was so pathetic. I don't know why he would be doing that. But I feel horrible that I just threw it in his face in front of you. He doesn't deserve that." She paused and started to cry again. "I just wanted him to be happy about last night and he wasn't. Then he was so mad, I don't know. I can't look at him. He's just going to hate me forever." Kim began to cry again.

Bob stared at the wall, his face as frozen as a marble sculpture.

The session went on and on. Jack tried to reassure them, but he couldn't get them to talk much more. They wouldn't even look at each other. He offered them another session that week, with the choice to come in separately or together. They said they'd let him know. He told them about how the Chinese character for the word "crisis" means both danger and opportunity. He told them about the couple that survived an even more dramatic breach of confidence.

None of it helped. They weren't listening to him. They were just waiting to get out of the room, away from him and away from each other. They seemed utterly helpless and alone.

After the session Bob walked rapidly ahead of Kim toward his car.

"What time will you be home tonight?" Kim asked his retreating back as she fished through her purse for her car keys.

Bob didn't look at her. His shoulders were hunched and his arms were folded tightly across his chest, as if he were holding onto himself. He mumbled, "I don't know. I might be late."

Kim went toward him and touched his arm lightly and said, "I'm truly sorry about what happened."

Bob turned his head away. "Don't worry about it. I'll be fine. Let's not talk about it, okay?"

"No, we have to talk about it. You and I. We should have talked three years ago, but I don't think it's too late now. I want to understand."

Bob barely knew where he was driving. Images of the session stung with shame. It was bound to happen sooner or later, Bob thought. Evans was probably shocked. I'll bet he thinks I'm a queer. I can't believe that she just said it right in front of him. I don't know if I'll ever go back there. Just the idea that he knows is bad enough.

"Christ!" Bob shouted as he drove by his exit. Then his anger released like the air out of a balloon. At least Kim seemed genuinely sorry. She really didn't mean to do it. He doubted that she was going to want to talk about it, though. But, if she does, what the hell?

IV

Ellen and Jack spent the evening working on their children's homework. Megan had a French test and Alex had some spelling words she was supposed to memorize.

"Pay attention, dammit, Megan," snapped Jack.

"Okay, everybody, let's change partners," Ellen said lightly while giving Jack a glaring, "Don't mess with me" look.

Jack pulled himself together, and the rest of the evening smoothed out.

Later, as Jack clambered over Ellen to get to his side of the bed, she said, "I took the hit on a call from your dad today."

"What was he up in arms about this time?

"Something about Dukakis standing in a tank with a helmet on looking like an idiot. He went on and on about it. Anyway, how did the presentation go today?"

"Actually it was fine. I got into it and they liked it. But I had a disaster session this morning. A couple that has been doing well just went up in smoke. I couldn't do anything about it."

"Is that why you were so irritable with Megan?" Ellen asked gently.

"Don't you start being the shrink. But you're right. I hate it when I feel like a beginning therapist all over again. I've been doing this for 16 years. You'd think I wouldn't be such a spaz. The couple I saw today might not even ever come back for all I know. I need some kind of R and R."

Ellen leaned over toward him. "How would you like me to be your comfort woman for the night, soldier?" Ellen said teasingly as she ran her finger along his jaw line.

"Nah, not tonight, hon. I'm beat. Maybe this weekend. Okay?"

"Well, that's just as well. I'm tired, too," Ellen quickly replied. She gave him a peck on the cheek and rolled over.

Jack lay awake in the dark. He reviewed the session with Kim and Bob. He couldn't sleep. He listened to the rhythmic sound of Ellen's breathing and the crunch of the cars going over the snow still on their street. Second thoughts and scenarios raced through his mind like storm clouds.

A full moon rising in the East shone outside his window. Its silvery light poured into the bedroom. Jack yanked down the shade and went back to tossing and turning. He wished he had taken Ellen up on her offer.

After dinner with Sarah and Bobby, both Kim and Bob started picking up the plates off the table as the kids scattered.

"I'll do the dishes," Bob offered.

"No, that's okay, you watch the news," Kim said.

"Really, I don't mind."

"Well, let's do it together then."

They silently worked around each other, sharing the same space while neither touching nor making eye contact. Each furtively scanned the other for hopeful signs.

Sarah bounced in. "Hey, guys, the teacher really liked the collage I put together of the Apollo mission."

"That's great," Bob and Kim said almost in unison.

"God, you guys are so stereophonic."

Bob and Kim smiled at each other.

Later, they lay next to each other in bed, waiting. Bob knew they had to talk about it, but he couldn't imagine what he was going to say.

Finally, Kim spoke into the darkness.

"I'm really sorry about today. I feel it was a terrible thing to do to you. No matter how mad I was, you didn't deserve it."

"Maybe it's for the best. We weren't getting anywhere not talking about it. But I just couldn't believe you would say it there. It really upset me that you said that in front of him."

"I know. It's actually none of his business. I never thought I would bring it up. He obviously was surprised. He seemed completely frazzled by it all."

"Yeah, I know. That part was almost funny. He didn't know what to say. You could tell he was rattled. I'll bet it was a first for him, in spite of all his experience."

"Does it make it more embarrassing that he's a man?"

"I didn't think about that. But maybe it was. I felt like it was my father or my brother sitting there. You know what they would think. Just the thought of them finding out was thoroughly humiliating. It makes me sick to think about it."

"Did you start, um, I mean, don't answer if you don't want to, but did you start doing it when you were a boy?"

Bob lay silently wondering whether he could or would answer Kim's question. Part of him ached with the wish to talk about all of it. On the other hand, there was a voice in his head screaming, "No! No! Don't! Watch out!" as if he were about to drive off a cliff.

Kim whispered, "It's okay, you don't have to."

"I want to. I really would like to. I just never ever thought I would talk to anybody about it, that's all. Ever since I was a little kid, I . . . , I felt so ashamed. Like I must be really weird. The truth is, I started this when I was 12. It was right after my mother died. I used to put on her things and, then, well, I don't know, then I would jerk off. I don't know why it was such a big turn-on."

"What did putting on her things make you feel like?" asked Kim. She reached for his hand under the covers. It had been a long time since Bob had spoken to her in such an open and trusting way.

"All kinds of feelings. I can't describe it. There was an incredible sexual charge. But it also made me feel calm—almost like I was in some kind of trance. That doesn't make any sense, but maybe somehow touching her things made me feel closer to her. To be honest, I've never thought about this before. I really missed her. At the end, they didn't even let me visit her at the hospital. I never even got to say good-bye."

Bob's body shook as he began to cry. Kim moved over to him and pulled his head to her breasts. She made soft soothing sounds and stroked his hair. She could almost imagine him as a boy, desperately seeking a way to hold onto his mom, using his mother's clothes almost in the way a toddler carries around a favorite "blankie."

After a bit, Bob pulled away a little and said, "I want to tell the rest."

"Are you sure?" Kim didn't want to push him too hard, but she wanted him to know she could listen. She hoped she could.

"Just say as much as you would like."

"I want it all out there. I'm sick of hiding."

"When I went away to college, I thought it was over. It hardly ever crossed my mind. I just chalked it up to kid stuff. But one time, after Bobby was born and I was home alone, you asked me to fold the laundry. I was just absentmindedly doing it when somehow—oh, this is hard to say—somehow, feeling your panties brought it all back to me. All of a sudden I found myself putting them on. I couldn't believe I would do that again. I was shocked how much it still turned me on. I was so ashamed, but it didn't stop me. Don't get me wrong, it's not like I did it all the time. After a while I began trying on more of your stuff."

"How could you even fit into it?" asked Kim, trying to restrain a smile at the thought. Bob wasn't a big man, but they weren't exactly the same size.

"Well, truthfully, with difficulty. I was always afraid that I would rip something. Some of it was actually funny. I can't believe I'm saying all this. But the first time that I put on one of your bras, I couldn't get it off. I could hear you and the kids coming in downstairs from shopping and I couldn't open the damn hooks in the back. I was panicked. I heard you coming up the stairs, so I quickly threw on a sweater and pants, just in the nick of time. I didn't get a chance to get the thing off until after you went to bed. That whole night I was terrified that you'd hug me and feel the straps. I think I even picked a fight with you so you'd keep your distance. I was so scared."

Kim chuckled out loud as she captured the image of Bob struggling with the bra hooks as she came up the stairs. "I don't mean to laugh, hon. Still, you have to admit it's a pretty comical picture. But what does putting on a bra do for you, anyway? Personally, I hate wearing bras." She paused before asking, "You don't want to be a woman, do you?"

"I knew you would think something like that. No, I don't think it's really about being a woman. But I still don't really know why I started doing it in the first place. It's all mixed up in my head about my mom. It just made me feel good. It was more than just a turn-on somehow. It was relaxing and made me feel better."

"Does it bring your mother back in some way?"

"I don't know. Maybe. Doing it made me feel less lonely, like she was almost still there. I know that really doesn't make any sense. I don't want to talk about her. I never even think about her."

"By the way," Bob said, pulling away from her a little, "you should know that, after you came in on me, I stopped doing it entirely. Not once in the last three years have I done it. Having you see me that way was the most humiliating moment of my life. I just decided it wasn't worth it."

"Do you still want to, though?"

Bob lay still. He knew the answer to her question, but he was afraid to say it. Kim took his hand. She knew his silence was the answer. Much to her surprise, she felt full of love and understanding. She felt the same kind of tender protective feelings she had when she helped him through their first few times together. A surge of erotic desire welled up in her. She leaned over to him and gently brushed his mouth with her lips. He put his arms around her, pulled her closer, and kissed her back, hard. As their bodies touched, she could feel his rigid penis between them. The intensity of his excitement aroused her even more. She pulled him to her. He held her tightly and kissed her with surprising ferocity. She returned his kiss in kind.

After a bit, she raised her head and said, "I love you."

" I love you, too. More than you'll ever know, and I'm so sorry."

"It's okay. It really is. Wait a sec. I've got to go put my thing in."

"I'm not going anywhere."

On her way back from the bathroom, Kim paused in front of her bureau, and then took out the pair of lacy black panties that came with the negligee. She couldn't believe she was about to do this for him. But it shouldn't be such a big deal, she reassured herself, just clothing. And it obviously meant so much to him. She smiled to herself. So what part does this come under—"for better and for worse" or "in sickness and in health"?

She climbed back into bed, snuggled up close to him, and said, "Here, why don't you slip these on?"

Bob shuddered. "No, I don't think I could."

"It's really all right. I understand."

"Thanks, but I. . . . "

She put her finger to his lips. "Ssssh."

They embraced again. They were suddenly floating, moving with each other in that awkward, graceful slow motion of space walkers.

QUESTIONS FOR DISCUSSION

1. What was the impact of Bob and Kim's family-of-origin experience on their intimate life, both in the early stages of their relationship and in the present?
2. What allowed Bob and Kim to have a different kind of sexual encounter at the end of the story? How did you feel about it?
3. How was what happened caused by the therapy, and was it a good outcome?
4. Was it inevitable that the cross-dressing come out in therapy, and was its exposure necessary for the treatment of the case?
5. Dr. Evans was upset about the session because it felt like it had been potentially destructive for the couple. Have you ever had a session that felt bad to you but that seemed to turn out well for your clients? Or vice versa? What are the implications about how we evaluate our sessions?
6. What are your strengths and weaknesses with treating sexual issues?
7. How did you feel about the cross-dressing behavior, and how do you address your counter transference responses to clients whose race, class, or sexual orientation may be quite unfamiliar to you?

MALIBU BARBIE
LOVES YOU

"Come on, now, it's getting close to naptime, Allybits," I say as gently as I can. None of my dreams about having a daughter included the nightmare of playing with dolls around the clock. I stand up and brush the lint off my rumpled work skirt.

"But, Mom, the Barbies aren't tired," whines Ally. "Look, Malibu Barbie is ready for the beach."

Ally holds up the impossibly endowed blonde in the sparkly pink bikini.

Where did she come from? I wonder as I kneel back down next to my four-year-old fashionista. How did I get such a girly daughter after having been a complete tomboy myself? I was going to grow up to be the Lone Ranger until my mother browbeat me into submission. I can still hear her exasperated tone when she pronounced, "Now Beth, you know girls don't play cowboys and Indians. You have to leave your brother's stuff alone. Why don't you play with your stuffed animals or your dolls?"

"I hate dolls!" I shouted back at her, and me yelling at her was always the last straw. It was okay for Johnny to lose his temper, but God forbid her precious daughter got mad. It wasn't ladylike. To this day my mother still believes in "sugar and spice and everything nice."

So here's Ally, Mom's revenge. Her room is fit for a princess with pink walls and matching pink ruffled bedspread covered with stuffed animals. Ally loves lacy frills, nail polish, party dresses, and her Barbies.

At least Peter and I shared the same image of what we wanted in a daughter. Peter certainly wasn't the typical urban Jewish intellectual. He's always been an aggressive outdoorsman, and right from the start he wanted to take Ally skiing, hiking, and sailing. I remember our first hike up Mt. Monadnock with Ally when she was only 12 weeks old. Peter carried her in his Snugly almost the whole way. She was wide-eyed and alert. When we got to the top, Ally set to squawking like a hungry eaglet, and I took her behind some rocks, unbuttoned my chamois cloth shirt, and pulled my noisy baby to me. Her mouth puckered in anticipation. A look of wonder and excitement shone in her eyes as she lifted her little head toward my breast. When she caught hold, her taut little body seemed to sigh into contentment. I leaned against the ancient granite and gazed out over the jagged expanse of the New Hampshire mountains and felt myself flowing into her. I was just drifting off, imagining myself as an Indian mother pausing in our wanderings hundreds of years ago, when Peter snapped a picture.

That Christmas, Peter's best present was that picture in a polished mahogany frame. The card said:

To the two best girls in the world—
We are the Three Musketeers. Remember, "One for all and all for one."
Happy Holidays and much love from the third one, Peter.

But, despite Peter and me, Ally had become this walking cliché of femininity.

"Don't worry. Once she gets into sailing she won't be so prissy," said Peter one night while we were discussing Ally's proclivities. So I suppose if we don't get back together, he'll be teaching her sailing on his own.

By the time I snap out of my reverie, Malibu Barbie's already at the beach and looking to meet up with Ken, who's exasperatingly late according to my babbling little narrator. How am I going to get her down for a nap without a big fight? Since Peter left she and I have both been explosive. Either one of us can be the match in the munitions factory. Sometimes I feel like I could hurt her. I know that's not true. But I feel it.

"Listen, sweetie, I know Barbie isn't tired, but she can rest at the beach while she's waiting, and you can take a nap too. Your mommy has to go downstairs and see her clients, and I'll be back before you get up. How's that?"

"No. I'm *not* tired. Just because you're a doctor lady doesn't mean you know everything. You don't know I'm tired!" Ally's face contorts into a ferocious scowl as she revs up for a major meltdown.

"You just can't make me late again," I warn, my voice rising to a shrill pitch. "We've been playing with these dolls for hours. I have to go, dammit. Get into your bed. *Right now!*"

I bend over to grab her. Ally's eyes open wide and her face turns white with fear. She leaps up and jumps into her bed, pulls the covers over her head, and starts sobbing.

Now look at what I've done. I kneel by her bed and try to hug her, but she slides away and then scrunches up into a little ball. "I want Daddy," she whispers.

"Allybits, I'm sorry," I say softly. "Please, would you like me to sing to. . . . "

I catch sight of her Little Mermaid clock on the nightstand. "Shit," I mouth under my breath. "I've got to run, sweetie," I toss back at her as I flick off the light and hurry downstairs toward my office.

"Hi, I'll be right with you," I say with my best professional smile to the Evans couple who are already in the waiting room. I slip into my bathroom. I need just a minute to pull myself together. Somehow I have to transform the wild-eyed raggedy bitch who just scared the hell out of her daughter into a calm, cool, and collected psychologist. I yank a brush through my straggly, dirty hair and put on a little fresh lipstick. I look haunted. It reminds me of the stricken look on Peter's face when he told me.

It started innocently enough, with one of our favorite Sunday afternoon rituals. Peter and I went on a long walk through Mt. Auburn cemetery with Ally playing hide-and-seek behind the headstones. It was one of those early spring days with a warm sun and soft blue sky. There were tiny green buds dotting the trees. I glanced at Peter as we walked along. He was strikingly handsome with his clipped salt-and-pepper hair; intense, almost black eyes; and distinguished jawline. He's stayed in what he calls "fighting trim." Meanwhile, I'm spreading out like pancake batter plopped on the skillet, I thought, as I inventoried my thickening waist, sagging breasts, and the newly arrived hint of a double chin. I never got my figure back after Ally.

We paused at various headstones and I played our old fantasy game about the lives of the men, women, and children long gone. I made up that Mrs. John Abbot probably had a nervous breakdown when she got the news from Gettysburg in 1863, and she was carted off to a sanatorium. After all, I bet she had five kids under 10 and she would have been only 28. Maybe her parents looked after the kids while she was convalescing. But she did go on to live until 1903. She never married again because here are the Abbotts, side by side.

Peter didn't play off my story with his usual wry humor.

And, of course, we stopped by my family plot where all the Hollingswoods have been buried for 100 years. There were about 40 headstones surrounding a marble bench that had our name engraved on it. The bench captured the essence of my mother and her family: elegant and smooth, cold and hard. Mother was able to disapprove totally of my whole life—me being a therapist, marrying a Jewish man, waiting so long to have children—with just a slight pursing of her lips and a sad shake of the head. Peter used to say I was every bit as much of a haughty Hollingswood as Mother was. Unfortunately, he had a point, but I always countered that at least I spoke my mind.

On the walk back to our Suburban, Peter was silent. Ally had raced up ahead.

"Peter, why aren't you talking?" I complained. "At least, talk to me about the campaign."

He shrugged his shoulders and sighed.

"Well, Beth, you know, I've got to get this analysis into Dukakis tomorrow about the debate mess. I'll be up until past midnight writing the damn thing and. . . . "

"Tell me again what it's about," I smiled in my best geisha-girl style, which usually softened Peter up since it played so well to his sense of self-importance.

"If you really want to know, our man blew it on that rape question about Kitty. He came across like an accountant crunching numbers rather than a husband talking about his wife. It's killing us. And I'm the one who's supposed to tell him."

"This must be so hard for you," I said and reached for his hand.

Peter didn't take it. He stepped back and looked away.

"Peter?"

He turned toward me. There were tears in his eyes.

My stomach knotted up.

"This is bullshit, Beth. What I really have to tell you, what I can't stand having to tell you, is that I've been seeing someone and, ah. . . . "

"What do you mean 'seeing?' . . . "

"Come on, Beth, You know what I mean. She's someone in the campaign. We've been traveling together. You don't know her. I'm so sorry, honey." His face twisted up in a mix of fear, guilt, and defensiveness. "I didn't mean to fall in love with someone else. It just happened and. . . . "

I stared at his scuffed-up brown loafers, holding my breath. And that's it? I thought. You say a few words and destroy our family as casually as squishing an ant under your shoe. But I didn't say anything. I'd be damned if I let him make me cry. When he mentioned our chronic problems in the bedroom, I wanted to punch him in the gut. I wanted to rip his face off. But I didn't. For once I was able to lock my mouth shut. I just turned and walked away.

I yank the brush so hard through my hair it hurts. Pull your self together; I scold the fuming woman in my mirror. I've got to focus on Jack and Ellen's situation. It would be good to see them after all these years. I think I saw them back in the early 1970s, before Peter and I had even met, when I had just started my private practice. God, I was so nervous back then.

They'd come in early in their marriage, when Jack was still in graduate school and before Ellen started law school. They were separated, and he was involved with another woman. Ellen was a fireball of rage and Jack was very frightened of her anger. God, what would Ellen think if she knew that now my husband was having an affair? Our work went well back then. I don't remember much, but they stuck it out.

Usually I can count on being a pretty good therapist even if my own life is a mess. I'd rather see clients than think about the little wad of misery upstairs, wanting her daddy and crying herself to sleep.

Jack's wearing khakis, a green sweater, and a corduroy sports jacket. He's tall and gotten a little pudgy, with receding brown hair. He still looks a little slovenly despite having become quite prominent as a family therapist. Ellen has kept her figure and her well put-together look, even though her face had softened and she wasn't wearing much makeup. Somehow she had managed to make full partner while insisting on only working four-fifths time. The first woman at Blake, Hall, and Seward to pull that off, she'd announced proudly.

Ellen sits in her old spot on the green sofa nearest my chair. I'm sure she's noted the cluttered mess on my desk. Jack settles into the safety of the big easy chair on the other side of the room.

"I'm sorry I'm a little late." I begin: "What brings you back?"

"Well, I guess I should start," says Jack, "I was the one that had the bright idea to come back."

"He wanted to come in on his own despite being Mr. Family Therapy," teases Ellen.

"She's right. I find this hard to talk about. I mean generally, I'm not feeling good about myself even though things are going well. I still don't feel like I measure up. But the real problem is that when Ellen tries to comfort me, I sort of freeze up. Particularly around intimacy and sex. I know it's kind of unusual for a man, but I'm pretty unresponsive. I call it the "Dead Battery Syndrome." I mean, the car's in great shape. It's just the battery, you know." Jack looks at me sheepishly.

"Do you believe him, Beth?" Ellen shakes her head at Jack, "Only a man would think of a description like that."

"It would be hard to find that diagnosis in the DSM, Jack," I join in.

"So now it's two against one, huh," he says, smiling a little defensively.

"I'm sorry, I was just teasing you a bit, one clinician to another."

He glances at me, smiling warily. "I suppose I should be used to it. I was always my dad's favorite target."

"Well, I don't want to sound like your dad. I don't remember much about him from our earlier work. What's the deal with him?"

He sighs and Ellen perks up. She must be thinking "bingo" in response to my opening up Jack's relationship with his father. My gut tells me to go for it.

"This may be a stretch, Jack. But what would you say was the most important moment you had with your dad when you were little?"

Jack pauses for a long time, looking out the window onto my yard.

"I don't remember much when I was little. Do you want any memory?"

"Sure."

"Well, this seems kind of dumb, but there was this one time when I was about four or five. I'd found this robin's egg in the backyard. I'd never seen one before. It was such a bright blue, so smooth and perfectly shaped, I was sure it was a magic egg. I hid it in my room because I didn't want anyone to tell me I had to give it back. At night, I would sneak it out of my bottom drawer and hold it my hand to warm it while I slept. I thought maybe a magic bird would hatch out of it."

Jack looks suddenly at Ellen and me and colors slightly. "We're not talking major trauma here. It's just that. . . . " He rubs his hand over his eyes.

"Go on, Jack," I say gently. I can see that Ellen is right there with him.

"Well, nothing was happening with the egg. I figured my dad would know what to do because back then I thought he knew everything. But he was still at sea on his ship and it would be weeks before he got home. I decided to wait for him anyway, no matter how long it took. I didn't tell anyone else.

"The night he came home was a big deal like always. Skipper, that's what we all called my dad, was in his dress whites, and Mom cooked a roast and my older brothers and sisters and I were spiffed up. We always had a parade inspection with Jonathan playing the pipes and all of us from tallest to shortest standing in a row."

"Anyway, he came in later to say goodnight and I showed him my magic egg. He held it in his hand for a moment and when I told him about warming it every night, he threw his head back and laughed. Then he tossed it to me. We weren't that far apart. I should have been able to catch it, but I," Jack paused, "but, I didn't. I dropped it on the floor and it cracked. I started to cry. Skipper just looked annoyed. He got up quickly and headed for the door. 'Lights out sailor, and listen, Jack, it's only a robin's egg; there's plenty more where that came from. And, hey, you're never going to make it in Little League if you can't catch.' "

"Some tragedy, huh?" Jack says, shaking his head, tears in his eyes.

"You wouldn't believe what a hard ass Skipper is," Ellen says to me, "He still treats Jack like that."

"Come on, Ellen, he's just. . . . "

"Just a sec, Jack," I jump in, "before you rush to his defense. Ellen's trying to be supportive."

Jack nods, but he's also retreated a little, just like he said he did in response to Ellen.

"It's happening right here. What are you feeling, Jack?"

Jack is gripping his fingers tightly in his lap. "I . . . I feel like she's going to be disappointed. That somehow her loving me won't make me feel better and then she'll get annoyed like my father would and. . . . "

"Hold on, Jack. Turn and look in Ellen's eyes right now. What do you see?"

Jack self-consciously looks into Ellen's eyes.

"Well?" I prod a little.

"I guess I see gentleness and love there."

"Is it different than how your dad looked at you?"

"I surrender, Beth, really, I get it," he says in a way that makes me wonder if I've pushed too hard.

Ellen jumps in, "You know, I'm nothing like his dad, but I do have to admit that I can be quite upset when Jack's not responsive to me. He's got a point."

Jack smiles at Ellen. He feels this support. It's funny how they seem to have a gentler, softer version of their old issues around Jack's fear of her anger. He's not as passive–aggressive and she's not as brittle. They've changed, and yet they are still have some of the same underlying patterns, just with the sharp edges sanded off.

By the end of the session, they're pretty close.

At least Jack was one man who would initiate therapy. He brought them in the first time, too. I wish Peter had suggested couple therapy before getting involved with this Nancy person. I asked him so many times. He always got mad and said, "People should handle their own problems." I'd accuse him of attacking my whole profession just because he was afraid. Then he'd say I'm just as controlling as my mother. I'd lose my temper. He'd lose his. We would rage at each other. End of conversation.

Now that everything's blown up, he's agreed to see someone. He says that it would be best for Ally, no matter what happens between us. Maybe it will help. Maybe it's too late.

I watch Jack and Ellen walk out into my driveway. They have a lingering embrace before they go their separate ways. I can't believe I'm feeling jealous of my own clients. I go back upstairs to check on Ally. I ease open her door and peek in, praying she's still asleep. Might give me a chance to dictate a few charts and get my act together. I've got to stop being so bitchy. None of this is Ally's fault.

I tiptoe over to the side of Ally's bed and just stand there for a moment, watching my little four-year-old, curled up and slurping on her thumb. Ally rolls over and I pull the covers back up to her neck. I lean over and kiss the curly tangle of blonde hair covering her forehead. She's just about the same age as Jack was in his story.

Damn.

The third ring of the phone jolts me and I hurry off to our bedroom.

"Hi," says the familiar voice, and I feel a rush of adrenalin.

"Are you busy?" Peter asks awkwardly.

I'm speechless. I bite down hard on my lip.

"Beth, are you there?"

Finally my normal composure kicks back in. "Of course, Peter, what can I do for you?" I say in my most cordial voice.

"Well, I was wondering if, you know, when I come to pick up Ally on Saturday, maybe we could all do something . . . ?"

"Like what?"

"Like maybe go on the swan boats. She always used to love that."

I can't breathe. Is this it—the opening my therapist and my friends all predicted? He'll be back, they said. Affairs blow over. Just give him a chance and don't get mad. You can get angry later, knowing full well how likely I would be to take Peter's head off given the opportunity.

"Beth?"

"Sorry, I was just trying to think."

"Well, I thought it might be fun."

"So is your lady friend unavailable or doesn't she like children?" I ask casually. Just the right tone, strong, but not too sarcastic.

"Please don't start. . . . "

"*Start*? Excuse me. You don't want me to start. What? A fight? Oh, of course, you don't want me to get mad. Why should I wreck a good thing? You just gave me a great invite and now I'm ruining it. Right!"

"Beth."

"Fuck off, Peter!" I slam the phone down. I want to smash it into the wall, but then I just burst into tears.

I throw myself on our bed and sob into my pillow like a teenager. I'm so mad I can't see straight. Naturally Peter will go and tell his shrink that, after all, he *tried*. Dammit! Damn him!

But I was the one who blew it. My goddamn temper.

"Mommy," came the little voice.

"Oh, Ally, I . . . " and then I start to cry again. Ally runs over to the bed and holds the Barbie up to my face. "It's okay, Mommy. Malibu Barbie says she loves you."

Great, now I've got my frightened daughter offering Malibu Barbie as an emissary to take care of me. What's wrong with this picture? I reach out and take the doll in my hand and look into Ally's worried and pleading blue eyes. I give Malibu Barbie a kiss on her forehead.

Ally smiles, climbs up on the bed, and lies next to me. "You know what?"

"No, what?"

"Barbie says everything is going to be okay," she pronounces and snuggles up to me.

As I take her in my arms, I notice the picture of me nursing Ally on the hike. Peter's card is still tucked in the frame on his bureau. My eyes fill again and I pull Ally even closer. It's frightening how much I need her.

But, hey, I'm supposed to be the grown-up and here I am hanging onto my little girl for dear life. I just wish that bastard would come home to us. What if I blew my one chance because of my stupid temper?

Suddenly, I am fully aware of the little four-year old body in my arms: the rise and fall of her tiny rib cage and her curly head tucked up under my chin.

I just want to blurt out the hard truth. Tell her I can't protect her from her father and I making a mess of our marriage, that I have no idea whether we'll be able to put back together the family she was meant to grow up in. I can't even protect her from myself and my stupid temper. All I can do is be here with her. I want to tell her everything, but I won't.

I give her a gentle little cuddle and whisper, "Yes, sweetie, and you can tell Barbie, she's right, it is going to be okay."

Ally gives me one of her sunshine smiles and then snuggles down with her head on my breast and pops her thumb in her mouth.

God, why couldn't I have just said yes to Peter and the damn swan boats?

QUESTIONS FOR DISCUSSION

1. Beth was able to be emotionally present and skillful with the Evans couple despite being very upset personally. In what ways did the session with the Evans couple have a positive and/or negative impact on Beth's interactions with either her daughter and/or her husband?
2. Beth is a therapist whose own life is in shambles. How do you react to her as she struggles with managing her anger with both her daughter and her husband? Do we hold greater expectations of her because she is a therapist? Do you hold yourself to a higher standard?
3. What kinds of crises have you had to manage in your personal life while practicing professionally? What helped you while going through those difficult times?
4. Both Jack and Beth are therapists having problems in their personal lives. How do the difficulties we have in our own relationships affect our clinical work? And how does our clinical work affect our relationships?
5. Beth is envious of her clients' closeness. Have you ever felt envious of your clients because they were doing better in their lives than you were in you own? What was that like?
6. Jack and his wife are in couple therapy. Have you been in therapy? Do you think all clinicians should have some experience in therapy? Why?

MAJOR GOATS

"They might as well've had me in handcuffs back there. It was just like a cop show. They were in the front seat making ridiculously small small talk and acting like we're going out to the mall or something instead of the stupid shrink's. And I was mushed in the back like a can of sardines just because they forget how tiny their Toyota shit box is and I'm not exactly their little boy any more. Anyway, I was dying for a smoke. So I rolled down my window.

"Then my mom whines, 'Jimmy, please don't put your window down. It musses my hair.' She was having one of her bad hair days."

B.J. and Wilson chuckled. They're a pretty good audience for my ongoing soap opera with my parents. They know the 'rents and I don't get along. They never come over to my house anymore. My mother used to serve them lemonade and talk to them like she's their friend and then I'd make a wisecrack or something and the next thing you know she'd be on my case right in front of them. It's all been different since we had to move here after my dad got laid off. In my old neighborhood, my house used to be Grand Central; everybody would hang out there back in the day.

Anyway, we were sitting in the caf with the classic Friday tuna noodle casserole and peas lunch. I was looking forward to telling them about what happened. I'm always trying to get a laugh out of them and last night was way over the top. I figured it would bust them up.

I'm actually still a little freaked out about the whole thing. But I wasn't going to let that get in the way of a good story.

So I scarf down my coke and continue.

"So get this. All I said was 'Yes, mother,' very politely.

" 'Don't use that tone with me!' she said.

" 'Bite me,' I whispered.

" 'Jimmy, I heard. . . . '

" 'Darlene,' said my dad, 'don't get into it with him.'

" 'Whose side are you on?' she snapped back.

" 'Don't go there, Dar. I just want to keep a lid on it 'til we get to whats'is name's office.'

" 'Great,' she said. 'What's the point in bothering to go to Dr. Evans if you won't even tell him to stop swearing at me? You never stand up for me.'

"Herrreeee they go, I thought and I relaxed a little back into my seat. They forget all about me when they're going at it about me."

That line gets a laugh out of B.J. and Wilson. But it was true. Yakking at me is about all they do. Usually my mom just makes a lot of noise and my dad doesn't give two shits. I could get away with murder as far as he's concerned. They're both pathetically afraid of me. Like I've turned into Frankenstein or something.

"So, anyway, guys, there they are yammering at each other and I'm chillin'. I was hoping maybe they'd spend the whole stupid meeting having this fight and I wouldn't be on the hot seat at all. Damn, that would have been cool. I figured afterwards I'd head on over to the Square and find you guys. You know, they actually bribed me into going to this dude by saying I could go out for a couple of hours afterward, even if it was a school night. They're so lame.

Anyway. That's why I had the weed on me in the first place. So then we get there and then the whole thing went crazy."

I pause for a little effect.

B.J. says, "Go on, man, tell us the rest."

Wilson and B.J. had barely touched their lunch and, believe me, if B.J.'s too distracted to eat you've got him hooked. B. J. is a big jelly doughnut of a kid. He's always smiling. He comes from this all-American family where everybody gets along and they're always doing family projects and shit. Like, they actually painted their house together. And they do these backpacking trips into the Canadian wilderness: just the five of them. B.J. complains about what his dad calls FFF (forced family fun), but Wilson and I know that secretly he really likes it.

Wilson, he's a runt. Puberty hasn't stopped at his house yet. And he never talks. He's as quiet as a snake and you never know what going on with him. His parents split up when he was little, and I've seen his stepfather rag on him and his mom. That guy is a certified prick, but Wilson never says boo about him. But you can just tell he feels bad about it. Him and B.J. have been best friends forever.

I joined up in seventh grade when we moved here. I hit it off with them. But I was still the new kid and well, by that time, I was what Principal Blaney calls an "instigator." You know the bit about peer pressure. Well, I was the "peer." They never would have gotten into dope if it weren't for me. I was always getting us busted. They'd get grounded and stuff and their parents blamed me. Okay, ripping off some CDs at the mall really was my idea, I admit. But I'm not that freaking bad. Now, they're not supposed to even be seen with me, for Chrissake.

My folks never do anything. Until last night: I don't really know what the hell's going to happen now.

"So, anyway, guys, we're all lined up in a row on this shrink's sofa like we're sitting in a church pew with me in the middle and, of course, Madam Motormouth starts right off ragging on me to the Evans guy about my 'negative attitude.'

"Well, the first thing the man said was 'I can't remember whether you would rather have me call you Jim or Jimmy?'

" 'Whatever floats your boat, man,' I said, like I'm supposed to care what the headshrinker calls me.

" 'Why don't you go sit in that chair,' he pointed to the other side of the room, 'You still look a little squished there between your folks.'

" 'Whatever,' and I slide over to the other chair. This is the third time he's started off by making me switch seats. Musical fucking chairs.

"Then he turns to the 'rents and tells them to figure out what they want to talk to me about.

"The next thing you know they're arguing like in the car. Mom starts complaining about my dad being such a wimp. She's always on his case since we moved here. I stretched out in my seat to watch the show.

"Then the shrink said, 'Let's deal with something that's going on right now.'

"My mom jumps right in and says with this big know-it-all look on her face like she's Agent 007 or something, 'Jimmy's got some pot in his jacket pocket. I saw him get it out of his drawer just before we left. How's that for something going on right now, Doctor Evans?'

"And I'm thinking, oh shit, I'm screwed.

"The next thing you know she's in my face with her hand out, screaming at me to give it up.

"I don't say a goddamn thing and the shrink told her to sit down and work out a plan with Dad about what they're going to do about it. She looks at him like she thinks he's the nut.

"So somehow the shrink and them figured my dad should lean on me. I don't know why, maybe because it's always my mom who's leading the charge and that hasn't done anything. Maybe the shrink's trying to shake things up.

"So my dad gets up and he's right in front of me saying 'Give it up, Jimmy.'

" 'Fuck you,' I said."

" 'You said that to your father?' cut in B.J., looking like I just broke one of the Ten Commandments or something.

" 'Yeah, well, this is therapy so you're supposed to be able to say what's on your mind.' Anyway, it really pissed him off. All of a sudden, he grabbed at my jacket like he was going to take my stash, so I pushed him and he pulled me out of the chair and then all hell breaks loose. I tried to run out of there and he grabs onto me. Unfucking believable. Where did he suddenly get the big *cojones*? The shrink gets up quickly and starts to separate us like he's a referee or something. This Evans dude is talking as cool as a cucumber like this kind of shit is an everyday occurrence. Things start to settle down when all of a sudden my mother grabs at my pocket from behind. Like now they're a WWF tag team and the whole thing is going insane."

B. J.'s laughing so hard he snorts his milk up his nose. "So then what?" he chokes out.

"Well the shrink sort of took over. First he orders my parents to get their hands off me. Which was a good thing because I was about to coldcock my dad in his face. Then he turns to me and says, 'Give me the stash, Jim, or else I'm calling the police.'

"So I gave him the damn bag and booked it out of there."

"Dude, this is truly whacked," says Wilson. Suddenly I look around and see the kids at the nearby tables are all staring at us. Even bigmouth Allison is right there. Then everybody's looking away like they're all concentrating on their food. Shit. This damn story will cover the school by the end of the day. Just what I need.

Just then the bell rings and the whole caf jumps into action, kids stuffing the rest of their food in their mouth and picking up trays.

"Wait, Jimmy, you've got to tell us what happened after that. Are you grounded for life or what?"

"Grounded is only half of it. Listen, I've gotta go." I grab my book bag and start sliding out of there. "I'll catch you guys tomorrow. My dad's leaving his new job early to pick me up and take me straight home. And, hey, don't bother with calling tonight. They've taken away everything, phone, TV, my boom box. Everything. I'm in total lockdown."

"Whoa, that's harsh," says Wilson.

"Yeah, they searched my room and found the rest of my stash and my pipe, too. I'm totally busted. My dad said he's going to start taking me for piss tests, too. Said I couldn't even get my permit until I was clean for six months."

"Man, this blows major goats," says B.J., still chuckling.

B.J. and Wilson head toward their math class.

"Yep, major, major goats. I'll see you guys." Then I turn toward Smathers's class.

"Man, do you believe that shit?" snickers Wilson, and I see him elbow B.J. in the ribs and hear them laughing together again as they stroll down the hall.

Suddenly telling them all this stuff doesn't seem like such a bright idea. The word is going to get out; everyone's going to think I have a messed up family and I'm a total psycho. This sucks. I should have kept my mouth shut. I don't know why I tell Wilson and B.J. this stuff about my family. They don't really give a rat's ass about me. They'll just party on. If I didn't supply the dope, they probably wouldn't still hang out with me anyway. My best friends. I'll bet by the weekend they'll forget why I'm grounded.

Smathers's class is all about Hamlet being and not being or something, but I swear everyone is sneaking peeks at me. Now, I know they're really not doing that. If I thought they were, then I would be a psycho for sure. And I'm really not. At least not certifiable anyway. I just want to get the hell out of here. This day is getting worse by the minute. I hate this stupid school. I want to go home. It's just as well my dad's picking me up because I don't want to hang with those guys anymore today. They'd want even more details. And the whole thing doesn't seem so funny now. I had a fight with my parents at the shrink's office. That *is* nuts.

And I still don't get what was up with my old man. How did he end up being the tough guy? He hasn't ever laid a hand on me except when we were playing around and roughhousing when I was a kid. We were really buds back then. We collected baseball cards, he taught me poker, and he let me play with the toy soldiers that he had collected when he was a kid. We even built a tree house together. Mom was always complaining about the testosterone overload in the house and that it was like having two sons. I thought it was cool.

But all the good times ended when he got fired and they said we had to move close to my mom's family for "support." I know that mom's family thinks Dad's kind of a loser. Even my Mom was probably thinking that. Thank God, he's got a job on his own now.

But, anyway, when we got home last night, all of a sudden he's gone drill sergeant on me with all these new rules and stuff. I don't know what the shrink said to them after I left, but he was different.

And he wasn't even being mean about it. He was just doing it. And my mom let him, too. She kept her big mouth shut for a change.

Smathers is talking about Yorick and his skull when the bell finally rings. I slip out into the hall and make a run for the men's room. Figure I'll wait there until the place clears out. I'd just as soon not run into anybody, and, honestly, I don't want people seeing me picked up by my dad like I was in sixth grade or something. This whole thing has gotten too weird.

At least I don't have to ride home on the bus.

QUESTIONS FOR DISCUSSION

1. What are the family dynamics that seem to be in play that might have contributed to Jimmy's substance abuse?
2. What was the therapist trying to do in this session, and was it effective? Why?
3. In what ways is Jimmy affected by the session?
4. Have you or anyone you've known been in family therapy when they were an adolescent? What do you imagine the experience is usually like for a teenager?
5. How would you describe what happens to Jimmy in the course of his telling the story to his friends?
6. What was difficult about your own adolescence and how did you get through it?

SPLIT ROCK GORGE

I

It's 7:55 A.M.—just five more minutes. Ann is sitting at her vanity carefully applying her eyeliner. She stares at her perfectly made-up self in the mirror and then pours the amber liquid into her glass. Just one more finger of Glenlivet. She thinks of the empty calories and the extra pounds she's put on in the last few months. Not good. Her weight has been 128 ever since she graduated from Smith, and after each child she fought her way back to it. I have to get back to running, she promises herself as she raises the glass to her lips. She would be good later. She takes just a little swallow. The last thing she wants is to be slurring her words when she talks with Dr. Evans. So far he has no idea how much she drinks, even though she's confessed to occasionally having a wee bit too much. He certainly didn't need to know about her allowing herself this morning treat.

Somehow she had already told Evans too much—secrets she'd buried long ago from when she was a little girl, secrets she swore she'd never tell and mostly had forgotten: like about her older brother, Dave, and playing "The Game," and seeing her mom and Mr. Dolan doing it right there in the living room when she got home from school early, and her father barking at her to take her pants down and bend over as he lurched back and forth and tugged his belt off his slacks. He did that even when she was older and it got even more embarrassing. Never mind the stinging blows that followed.

The therapy started simply enough. Her internist sent her to Dr. Evans because she seemed so tense. Dr. Phelps thought her anxiety might be might be contributing to her migraines and stomach problems. It had never occurred to Ann that she would need therapy because, after all, wasn't she a star "soccer mom," member of the Weston PTA, and a volunteer at Newton–Wellesley hospital? She was a good wife, good homemaker, and good mother. She shouldn't need to be in therapy.

Ann began getting the headaches when her daughter, Eliza, turned eight. She became obsessed with worries that something bad would happen to her little girl. She smothered her with anxiety about everything from catching colds, to wearing seatbelts, to the dangers of strangers. Despite being a very sweet little girl, Eliza would sometimes whine with exasperation when Ann insisted on her wearing another layer of clothing or would not allow her a play date with any friends whose parents might not supervise them closely enough.

"It's just going to be easier if Jennifer comes over here," Ann would say. "We'll make brownies."

"But, Mom, Jennifer always comes here. She thinks you don't like her parents."

"Now, honey, it's not that I don't like the O'Donnells. It's just that they let Jen watch way too much TV with all that violence, and I'm not at all sure her mother wouldn't think it was fine to slip out and run an errand, leaving you two all by yourselves.

"But Mom. . . . "

"No buts about it, or you can go to your room and play by yourself."

Eliza glanced pleadingly at her father, but he just rolled his eyes.

John was no help to Ann. He accused her of being neurotic and overprotective. She stopped talking about it and kept her worries to herself. That only seemed to make things worse. That's when the ferocious headaches and waves of nausea started.

More and more she retreated to the safety of her room. She'd pull down the shades, unplug the phone, and put on her nightie. Her doctor had given her some pills for the migraines called Fioricet. They helped a little, but Ann discovered they were much more effective when washed down with a few gulps of Scotch. She kept her bottle in her sweater drawer and was very careful to use it only medicinally.

After she took the pills, she'd put in earplugs and cover her eyes with a sleep shade and in the perfect black silence she could disappear. She dozed, sometimes sleeping, sometimes just floating as if she were an eagle riding the thermals high above the pasture, sometimes remembering herself as a little girl peacefully drifting around in her inner tube in their backyard pool, happy to be all alone.

Ann looks at the clock by her bed: 7:57. The check-in phone call from Evans seemed like a good idea when he offered it. It was kind that he was worried about her. But this therapy business was not making things better.

Somehow Dr. Evans had made her tell him things. Not exactly made her. It's just that he had these kind eyes and gentle manner. He really wanted to get to know her. Nobody had ever bothered before. John certainly had stopped being very interested a long time ago. After the kids came they had drifted into a nightmare fifties cliché: John, the workaholic, and her, the happy homemaker. John could care less about what happened in her day and, honestly, she wasn't all that interested in hearing about the high-flying deals he was making all over the country.

Ann got up from her stool and carried her glass over to her bedside table next to the phone. At least she and John didn't fight. And he never laid a hand on her. That was a very good thing.

When Evans asked her about what her family was like growing up, at first she maintained that everything was fine, just fine, but slowly things began to tumble out of her mouth. The first thing was about her dad and mom drinking and them fighting deep into the night.

Months ago, in the middle of a freezing day in January, she remembered sitting in his office in his big stuffed easy chair and screwing up her courage to ask him bluntly, "How is dredging up all these bad memories about my childhood going to help?"

She was afraid he'd be offended by the question, but Dr. Evans smiled at her. "Actually, Ann, there's no easy answer. Sometimes when we bury bad memories and feelings from back then, they often are what causes the intensity of our stress in the here and now. Sometimes talking about them allows us to truly let them go. Let's try it a little and see how it goes. We don't have to talk about anything you don't want to."

Ann looked at him tilting back in his office chair with his hands folded over his ample lap. His casual look, in his crew neck sweater and khakis, and his wrinkled brow and big brown eyes seemed inviting and safe enough.

"Well, I've told you there was a lot of drinking and fighting, but that's not the worst. My bedroom was right next to my parents', and I'd have to hear the most awful things. He'd call her names like whore and dumb . . . , well, other four-letter words, and she'd scream back at him things about how he couldn't get it up and couldn't last when he did."

She looked at Evans with tears in her eyes: "I didn't even know what they were talking about but whenever Mother said something about his, you know, capabilities, Dad would just go off and start smacking her until she pleaded for him to stop. Then there would be squeaking and grunting noises and then silence. Then I could go to sleep."

"What was that like for you, Ann?"

"It didn't really bother me. After all, by the time I was Eliza's age, I was kind of used it, you know. I would just pull the pillow over my head and cover my ears. Sometimes I could even fall asleep before they were finished." She felt oddly proud to report that to Evans.

The next session she decided to tell him about "The Game." She wore her royal blue suit, a maroon silk blouse, and her mother's real pearls for that session. She wanted to look her best.

In his office, she perched on the edge of her seat with her back ramrod straight and her knees pressed together.

"You seem tense today, Ann. What's going on?" asked Evans.

She sat still for a while. Then she looked at him hesitatingly.

"There's more that happened back then but it's really embarrassing to talk about. It started when I was about Eliza's age. My brother, Dave, was probably about 11. He started coming into my room when the parents were fighting. He'd be mad that they were making all this noise. He hated Daddy because Daddy used to beat on him almost every day—much more than me. Dave said he was worried about me. So he took me to his room so that he could "protect me" and let me sleep in his bed.

"At first, it felt really good. I felt safe and we would kind of cuddle up together and whisper about how much we hated our parents and were afraid of Daddy. He promised that he would protect me from Daddy even if it meant taking more beatings himself. He told me to imagine that someday I would be a grown up and have a home of my own and then everything would be all right."

Ann stopped and looked out the window at the gray sky. She turned back to Evans and said brightly, "Well, looks like more snow."

"Is there more to tell, Ann?"

She nodded her head "yes" and bit her lower lip. She looked down. "One night we were under the covers and he said, "Do you want to play soldiers?"

"What's that?" I asked.

"And he took my hand and placed it on his thing."

"See. He stands at attention just like a soldier."

I froze. I didn't want to make him mad at me. I knew we were doing something bad. He was breathing hard and whispering things like "Go ahead, rub him. Squeeze him hard."

Ann paused. Suddenly all her feelings drained out of her. She didn't feel like she was going to cry. She just felt as limp as a rag doll. She didn't want to talk anymore. She just wanted to go to sleep. She closed her eyes.

Evans leaned toward her and said, "Ann?"

She opened her eyes and looked at him. "So I masturbated him until he came. I mean, it wasn't like he really did anything to me. He never touched me. He wouldn't have wanted to hurt me. Besides, he wasn't even interested in what I looked like down there. He just wanted me to do his "soldier." That's what he called it, "playing soldiers." Then he started calling it "The Game." It went on for a long time. He had me do it whether the parents were fighting or not and even when we were home alone.

She smiled defiantly at Evans and said, "Well, there you have it. I jerked off my brother for a couple of years until he finally got a girl his own age to do it. And that's my big secret."

Evans talked to her quietly about how harmful and confusing it can be to have this kind of experience, but Ann wasn't listening. She had floated away.

It wasn't until after Evans got her to tell about "The Game" that all of these memories began to be too much for her. She liked the feeling of being listened to and telling her secrets. She began to rely more and more on her time with Evans. At least with him there would be some morsel of help and hope. During their therapeutic hour, she would feel held and understood like she never had before, and yet in the car ride home she would feel utterly alone.

Worst of all, Ann felt like more happened when she was little but she couldn't remember it. And she didn't want to. Sometimes when she was lying in bed she felt a crushing weight pressing on her body. And she couldn't breathe. But then it would go away. She didn't want Evans probing around with that. And she had barely hinted at half of what she was doing at home. She didn't want to scare him away, so she didn't tell him too much about the drinking and the additional Valium she'd convinced her internist to prescribe for her. She was very careful never to appear drunk. John didn't even notice the smell. Eliza asked her once, "What's that funny breath mint smell, Mom?" Ann smiled sweetly. "It's a butterscotch candy."

Ann spent more and more time in her room and needed more and more Glenlivet to rest. She couldn't quite tell Evans how bad it was. He was already worried that she had stopped going to her PTA meetings and her physical symptoms were worse. And when she told him that she couldn't perform the usual Saturday night routine with John, she left out how mad he was and that he told her that her stupid shrink was making her worse. Evans actually suggested that maybe she and John should see somebody together, which was the last thing John would ever do.

At least with Dr. Evans she knew that he really did care. It was his idea to offer to touch base while he was away on his trip. He even asked if she ever had suicidal thoughts.

"Of course not," she said quickly. "I could never do that to my children." She decided she'd better convince Evans she was doing better, because she was beginning to be bothered by precisely those kinds of thoughts. She didn't want him to put her in a hospital, but she wasn't as good at pretending as she used to be. She could no longer float away. More and more her thoughts returned to her childhood bed, the yelling, the hitting on the other side of the wall; when father went after her and Dave with the belt; and then the nights having to play with Dave's eager pathetic soldier.

More and more she was back there. More and more she thought about doing whatever it took to make the feelings go away. She couldn't soar like an eagle anymore. She felt like a terrified vole in an open field with a circling shadow overhead.

She looked at the clock next to her bed: 7:59. She took one more sip.

II

The roar of Split Rock Gorge warns Jack and Ellen that they're close. Their path winds through the towering Scottish highlands on the Isle of Skye. The root and rock strewn path is so narrow they're hiking single file toward the sound.

Ellen hiked into the Cuillin mountains three miles yesterday to see the gorge while Jack was giving his seminar. It was a primeval sight. The mountain stream sliced through 80 feet of solid granite. At the base of the cliff, the water thundered through the narrow cut over a jumble of boulders. Standing on the rickety wooden bridge across the gorge and looking down into the water gushing beneath her, Ellen was acutely aware that this mountain stream had been slicing though this rock for thousands of years. She felt small and insignificant. She found the wild and roaring stream strangely serene.

Now she's taking Jack to see it with her. It was well worth a second hike in; they didn't do enough stuff like this anymore since the kids came along. Beth had pushed them into taking some time off by themselves. This was the first time Ellen had been able to get away from the office to accompany him on one of his workshops. August was always their slowest month, and the kids were with her mother.

Ellen watches out for the nettles and poison ivy mixed in with the heather and warns Jack behind her. She's glad the kids aren't with them. Too many worries. But she's worrying about Megan anyway. She's convinced that her precocious 13-year-old is at risk for getting in way over her head with boys. Megan had always been such a trusting, innocent, and affectionate little girl. Unlike Alex, who, at eight, was the neighborhood tomboy—wiry, strong, and better at baseball than most of the boys on the block, Megan had always been the shy, sensitive one, tuned to every emotional nuance around, anxious to please. Now suddenly her body had blossomed and she radiated sensual energy. Overnight her baby had turned into a femme fatale wearing skintight tops and skirts that were up to here. Last week she even began lobbying for pierced ears.

"Almost there," she says to Jack.

Jack grunts back.

Ellen reassures herself that she survived her own provocative phase that drove her mother up a wall, too. She spent hours in front of the mirror and even surreptitiously stuffed her bra. At least Megan didn't have to resort to that, she thought with a slight twinge of jealousy. God, it must have been so obvious to my mother. She reddens.

"Hurry up, Jack," she calls back.

Ellen spent her whole life moving away from that kind of pinup girl version of femininity. What would happen when Megan's date started sulking because she was resisting taking care of his "needs"? Or maybe Megan would be the one consumed by her own desires? Times had changed.

Ellen pushes back a branch of a bush that blocks the trail and then holds it so Jack can come through. She's still lost in her own thoughts. Worrying about Megan and boys leads her back to Larry Gill and the countless hours she spent freezing behind the glass at the hockey rink. She'd stand there in the snow in a short skirt, with bare legs and wearing penny loafers. Her only concession to the cold was to have her face wrapped in his blue and white school scarf. As she followed each of his liquid moves up and down the ice, she'd shuffle back and forth her with her arms clasped tightly together and her breath swirling around her like cigarette smoke.

She suddenly remembers the bus ride home after the dance, when Larry's left hand snaked under her coat and caressed her breast. He leaned over to her and brushed her cheek with his lips. "I just want to be with you," he murmured.

The image of that night surges through her. No wonder she's worrying about Megan.

Jack watches the ripe swing of Ellen's hips in front of him and remembers following her 20 years ago across the quad. Before they even met, he had noticed her rear end and the easy rolling motion of her walk. He's surprised to be feeling exactly the same way now. Despite time and children, Ellen had stayed in very good shape.

Remembering Ellen and their college days stirs Jack up. He looks at his watch. They have a half an hour before the phone check-in with Ann. If he could end the call on time, they'd have 45 minutes before they went on the tour of Dunvegan Castle. Maybe Ellen would be up for a little fooling around. They'd been in Scotland for two days and they hadn't done anything yet. Maybe she'll be interested.

The path widens. Now the sound is deafening but they still can't see the gorge. They're beginning to walk down.

"You know, Jack," Ellen shouts at him as he catches up, "I think we're going to have to rein Meggie in a little. I'm worried about. . . . "

"This is why you dragged me out here, to talk about Meggie?" Jack teases.

"No, seriously, I think she might be a little too. . . . "

"Come on, honey. She'll be okay," Jack interrupts. "She's always been a solid kid and this stuff about looks, clothes, bodies, and boys seems pretty developmentally normal."

Jack didn't say how he worries in a different way. Meggie was always his cuddlebug, but now it's different. She still wants to sit on his lap and snuggle, but he's acutely aware of her ripe, full female body draped all over him, and is shocked by the occasional surge of his arousal. Recently, he had taken to gently disentangling her from him while they were watching TV on the couch, making sure he wasn't walking down the hall in his underwear, and chidingly telling her to put some clothes on when she pranced into their bedroom in just a baby doll nightie and bikini underpants. Jack didn't want a prude for a daughter, yet her surprisingly nonchalant ease with her own body made him just as nervous as Ellen, for slightly different reasons. Megan's little sister, Alex, was still his pal; they could throw the ball around or do puzzles, even dolls. He wondered if it would get just as tricky with her when she went through the whole thing.

"Jack, are you listening? I hate being pushed into the matronly role of having to scold her about boys and their urges. I'm beginning to sound like my mother. Will you talk to her about how boys will treat her if she keeps strutting around dressing the way she does? I'm beginning to wish she'd go for the 'grunge' look. At least that would cover her a little."

"What? I'm sorry, sweetie. I wasn't completely listening. I was distracted the whole walk by the sway of your sweet rear end. You know our daughter isn't the only sexy female in the house."

Ellen turns from the river and looks at him. His smile is playful and cute. Suddenly she feels young. She blushes. It's been a while since Jack's been flirtatious with her. "Oh, don't be silly," she says, while lowering her gaze.

Jack reaches for her and pulls her close. Then he cups her face in his big hands and gently brushes her nose with his nose, an Eskimo kiss from their courtship days.

Ellen puts her arms around his neck and kisses him: a soft, sensuous kiss, her tongue seeking his.

Jack shifts his weight to fully return her embrace and stumbles slightly over a root.

Ellen laughs, "Well, maybe it's not just me that's too old for a little outdoor necking. Is this too strenuous for you, my dear?"

Jack laughs back while holding her tight around the waist and pressing into her abdomen a little. "I don't know, maybe I'd be better at this lying down. I'll race you back to the room."

"But what about the gorge?"

"Screw it. It'll be there for the next thousand years. We'll catch it in another lifetime."

"But I really wanted to see it with you." Ellen reaches for his hand. "Come on, we'll still have time."

"No. I can't do the gorge and make mad, passionate love and still be on time for my check-in appointment with my client."

"God, Jack. I forgot about that. Why did you have to schedule it in the middle of the day, anyway?" She pouts like a teenager. Then she smiles mischievously, "I've got it. Let's still go down to the gorge. When we get back for your damn call, you can lie on the bed and talk to her. Meanwhile I'll just quietly unzip your pants and show you a really good time."

Then she boldly reaches over and cups his crotch in her hand and smiles seductively.

"Now, Ellen, stop." But Jack doesn't want her to. He's surprised and delighted with Ellen's playfulness. He never knows when to expect this side of her. Sometimes she's the all-business Boston lawyer, and sometimes she comes on like a sultry babe. The few sessions with Harney helped him feel less on the spot when she was the initiator. Today, he's right there with her. But then he thinks of Ann.

"Damn," he sighs heavily, murmuring, "You know I can't take you up on that offer. This woman's in a real crisis."

"I was just kidding, Jack. Don't lecture me. I just think it's a pain, that's all." Ellen steps back a little and looks away with her lips pursed.

Jack doesn't want to wreck the sexy mood between them. He pulls her back into his arms and says with mock seriousness, "Now listen up here, counselor, I've got a counterproposal. When we get back, you take a hot bubble bath, I'll do the phone call and I'll end it right on time, then I will do you with no strings attached. You just get to lie back and enjoy it. I won't be like one of those greedy guys you're so worried about trying to get into Meggie's pants. It'll be my gift to you to make up for the phone call. And we won't be late for the castle tour."

"Really. What about you?"

"I'll be okay. Don't you know that it's only a myth that men die from blue balls?"

"Well, that's sweet. I accept. But let's go take a look at the gorge from the bridge first. The thought of all that rushing water underneath me turns me on."

"What?"

"Oh, you men. You don't understand anything."

III

Jack lies back on the bed near the phone. Ellen is in the shower, singing an old Beatles song, "Ob-la-di, ob-la-da, life goes on bra, la-la, how the life goes on. . . . " Jack smiles. It's been a long time since he heard her singing. He suspects that his altruism may be generously reciprocated in the next few days.

Jack looks at the clock: 12:59 GMT, 7:59 A.M. her time. Ann will call right on the dot of eight. He imagines her looking at her clock, waiting. His stomach tightens in anticipation of the half-hour check-in session. He knows she's having a hard time with his being on vacation. This check-in phone call will be just a drop in the bucket for her.

Jack's also worrying that Ann isn't really telling him everything that is going on. Once he thought he caught of whiff of alcohol on her breath. Opening up her trauma history actually had seemed to make things worse. The sessions went okay, but who knows what's really going on. He'd finally surrendered his idiotic pride and contracted for some supervision when he got back. At least he knew enough to know that he needed help.

An ocean away, it's 7:59. Ann looks at the telephone number on her notepad. She forces herself to breathe. She counts down the seconds. Slowly she picks up the phone and dials the number.

"Skiboost House. May I help you?"

"Could you please connect me to Dr. Evans' room? Please."

Jack picks up the phone on the first ring. "Hello, is that you, Ann? Right on time."

"Hi," Ann says. Then there's a long silence.

"I know this is hard, Ann," Jack says.

"I don't know what to say. I guess it has been kind of hard," she mumbles. She has her glass in hand. Then she pauses again. She takes another sip.

"It's okay, Ann," Jack breaks into the silence. "Take your time."

QUESTIONS FOR DISCUSSION

1. The world of the therapist and the client are clearly quite separate. What do you think about the therapeutic relationship between Evans and Ann?
2. In what ways is it helpful and/or harmful?
3. Ann's remembering her trauma history seems to be making things worse. How would you treat Ann differently?
4. How does a therapist balance his or her personal and professional life when treating a potentially self-destructive, very vulnerable client?
5. Have you had experience working with trauma survivors, substance abusers, and suicidal clients? What are your strengths and weaknesses working with this population? What's most difficult?

2002

14 Years Later

DRESS-UPS

Elbows bent backward into angel's wings, Sarah Dunbar carefully tugged the zipper up the black silk Chanel sheath that her mom always wore to funerals. It seemed fitting to her to wear it today, and she was pleased she could squeeze into it. Her mother had been a determined size 8, and Sarah had always been a relaxed size 10. But, during these last few months, when she had eaten mostly bowls of cereal and popcorn and furtively taken up smoking again, she'd dropped 10 pounds. As she smoothed the dress down over her hips, Sarah wondered what size her mother had been near the end. Maybe a four?

Two days ago was the last time she had seen the thin wraith of her mom, her body barely making a shape beneath the sheets. Toward the end Sarah recoiled from looking at her mom's skeletal face sunk into the pillow. But Sarah had been there day and night: making idle chatter, swapping old stories, or watching TV, and toward the end, mostly silent. While her mom dozed, she watched the shaft of sunlight play across the room, reflecting off the white walls, the stainless steel tubing of the bed, the dials of the heart monitor, and the IV stand. She got so she could see the light sneak steadily across the room. Sometimes she sat, eyes closed, her hand resting lightly on her mom's dry birdbone hand. She patted it tenderly, as if tapping out a Morse code message over a great distance. *Don't - leave - me - I - love - you.*

Her tears began again. She grabbed her hairbrush and pulled hard on her mane of unruly auburn hair. But there was no escape. The pull on her roots flooded her with memories of her mother gently working out her snarls. "Sarah, honey, I don't know how you do it. I send you off every morning with a fresh, clean head of hair and you come home wearing a bird's nest. I swear someday I'm going to find a baby robin in there."

That always made her laugh.

She looked at the dark circles under her eyes and reached for her mother's makeup kit for a little concealer. She found some Cover Girl foundation that she smoothed on.

Not bad she thought, considering she never wore makeup except for maybe a wedding or something like this. She brushed on some mascara: It was like playing dress up.

It reminded her of that day in the attic when she had just turned seven.

It was dark and musty. Through the small window came a thin shaft of light filled with floating bits of golden dust. The attic was off-limits, her mom said. It was too dirty and too dangerous. Too many exposed nails and possible splinters.

Sarah sneaked into the attic and came upon an old trunk with her grandmother's name on a brass plate. Helen Bently Shaw. It was black with worn leather carrying straps. But it was locked. She looked over the dusty shrouded boxes and pile of old furniture, shrugged her shoulders, and was about to head back downstairs when she saw the key Scotch-taped to the side of the trunk. It was like finding a buried treasure. Inside she found neatly piled clothes reeking of mothballs. She rummaged through the silk, satin, and taffeta evening gowns. She pulled out one after another and held them up to her neck in front of an old gilt-edged mirror. Finally she picked out a straight black dress with long fringe at the hem and a spray of silver spangles across the bodice. She stripped off her blue jeans and T-shirt and put it on. It hung off her and the fringe trailed to the floor. Then she discovered a black-beaded silver cap that fit like a helmet, with a single ostrich feather jauntily swept back that reminded her of Robin Hood. She completed her ensemble with several long strands of white beads that hung down to her thighs.

Just as she stepped toward the mirror, teetering precariously on the shiny black patent-leather high heels, she heard her mother laughing, "My, my, look at our young flapper."

Sarah whirled around, tripped on the fringe of the skirt and collapsed in a heap. "I'm so sorry, Momma."

Her mother helped her up, wrapped her up in a big hug, and whispered, "It's okay, sweetie. You shouldn't have come up, but no harm's done. Besides, you look adorable in your grandma's Charleston dress. Your grammy was quite the party girl. I remember trying on this same dress when I was about your age."

"But I think I ripped it?"

"We can always sew it up; anyway, the next person who will wear it will probably be your daughter. I'll tell you what, let's go put some makeup on you and we'll surprise your father."

Her mom took her by the hand and carefully helped her down to the second floor.

Sarah was squirming with excitement. Her mother had never even let her try any lipstick on before and now here she was sitting at the vanity in her parents' bathroom with her mother working over her like a beautician. Her mom painted her face with eyeliner, lipstick, and a hint of blush.

Sarah was awed by her reflection. "I look all grown up, Mom. Am I pretty?"

"You sure are, sweetie. Let's test you out on your dad."

She called out to the master bedroom. "Bob, close your eyes. I'm going to present to you a miniature version of Greta Garbo."

Bob Dunbar put down the Sunday *Times*, closed his eyes, and said, "Ready when you are."

Her mother led Sarah right up to the side of the bed.

"Ta da!"

Bob opened his eyes. "Wow," he said. "Who is this young lady? You look just like your mother did when I first met her. How about a date?"

"You're a little old for her, don't you think. And besides, you're mine," her mother said with a chuckle.

The thought of her parents' being playful with each other yanked Sarah back to the mirror. She missed those days. She fought back tears.

She was late. Her dad would be there any minute. She dreaded seeing him—his awkward, eager-to-please look he always had on his face. He would try and butter her up by talking about how pretty she was and how much she was the spitting image of her mother.

The few times after the divorce that they tried dinner alone, his repartee was always the same. "You look great." "So, how's school?" "Umm, good menu. What are you going to have?" "Any special boys in your life?" "Is your mother okay?"

It was much easier when her brother Bobby was there. Dad acted more like he used to when they were little. She hated this tentative version of a father with his bizarre, supposedly secret activities. He must know that her mom had told her everything about what had happened. That certainly would explain his tentativeness around her. But she and her father had never talked about it.

Her mother told her three years ago. She had come into her room the first afternoon Sarah was back from Vassar in her junior year. Mom reached for her hand. Her eyes were red.

Sarah tightened right up. Her mother almost never cried.

"Sweetie, I've got some bad news." Her mom paused and looked away.

Oh, my God, she's sick, thought Sarah immediately.

"We were going to wait until you were through college, but we can't put this off any longer."

"Mother, what is it?"

Her mother plopped on the bed beside her. "Your father and I will be separating after the first of the year."

Sarah felt like she had been punched in the sternum. "Why? Why?" she stammered as her mind went blank. The idea of her folks splitting up was inconceivable. "You guys get along okay."

Her mom's shoulders sagged and she bowed her head. "Oh, honey, we've had our normal ups and downs like most couples, but … " She hesitated. "I think you're old enough to hear this, but I don't want you to tell Bobby. He looks up to your dad and he's a boy."

"Is Dad having an affair?"

Her mother stood up and walked over to her window that overlooked the backyard. "I wish he were. It would be simpler. I don't know how to say this."

Sarah stood up, walked over to her mother, and put an arm around her shoulder. "Just say it, Mom," she said softly.

"Your Dad likes to dress up in women's clothes," her mom said flatly.

Her mother's words didn't register at first. "Daddy? Daddy likes to put on women's clothes? Why?"

Her mother shook her head slowly and whispered, "I don't know, honey. He talks about having a female identity that he quote–unquote 'needs to explore.' "

"Does he do it all the time?" she asked.

"Seems like it, nowadays. He even goes out dressed to a support group with other men like him."

Sarah felt a rush of revulsion. Sarah had seen a lineup of crossdressers once on the "Jerry Springer" show, and the thought of her dad going off to be in a group of men like that was revolting. She wished that her mother hadn't told her. She looked out the window at the swing set that she played on and remembered her father steadfastly pushing her as she implored him to swing her higher and higher. The idea of him getting all dolled up like a woman gave her the same queasy *whoosh* she would get when she felt like she might fly right off the swing.

"How did you stand it?"

"I love your father. I tried to be understanding. We even went with our old therapist to a gender specialist that your dad had been secretly seeing on his own. I'll never forget it. Your dad met us there: all made-up and wearing a shoulder-length blond wig and my old green corduroy maternity jumper."

Sarah scrunched up her eyes. "I don't even want to think about this."

A rueful smile crossed her mother's face. "Well, of course, neither did I. He looked so strange. You know he's not that big and he was good at his makeup. So he looked more like a woman than I could imagine. And he wanted me to like him that way. But I just couldn't deal with it."

"How long have you known?"

Her mother sighed heavily and stared out at the big maple silhouetted against the fading light. "For more than 10 years. I tried hard to be compassionate. But, but. . . . " Her mom began to fight back tears. "At first it didn't seem like such a big deal. But I'm not sure I should tell you all this."

Sarah reached for her mom's hand and gave it a gentle squeeze.

"Well, okay, it started when you and Bobby were still little. I discovered that sometimes he liked to wear some of my things and I sort of went along with it. I mean, it was a very embarrassing and tender part of him. It even brought us closer for a while. I really tried to understand, but. . . . "

Her mom broke down into sobs and slumped against her. "But the more tolerant I was, the more he seemed to want to go further into it. When I told him enough was enough, he said he'd stop, but clearly he went back to hiding it. I didn't know what to do."

Sarah put her arms around her mother and held her tight. "It's okay, Mom. It's okay," she whispered as she realized it would never be okay again.

In the small yellow cottage that he had bought after the divorce, Bob Dunbar was getting ready. He rummaged around the back of his lingerie drawer. Tucked behind his breast forms, he found a pair of cotton Jockeys. It seemed fitting to dress in the old ways for Kim's funeral. She would have liked that small touch. He quickly pulled the underpants up his smoothly shaven legs. In the closet next to his dresses, he reached for an old business suit.

When he stepped outside gently cradling the three wrapped long-stem roses, a moist breeze was full of the pungent smell of the skunk cabbage in the backyard, always the harbinger of the coming spring. The crocuses were up and the green buds of the lilies were about to open.

He remembered that picnic their first spring, 30 years ago. They were down on the banks of the Charles celebrating their third month anniversary with Veuve Clicquot and brie. There she was with her wild tangle of blonde hair, brilliant blue eyes, and a splash of freckles over her nose. She sat on the blanket, leaning on her hand and brandishing her cup full of champagne. "Here's an Irish toast to you, Sir Robert. May the sun always greet you and the wind and rain be at your back or something like that and furthermore may you always be my knight in shining armor." Then she laughed and tossed off her drink.

Bob winced at the memory and reached for the car door. Some knight in shining armor he turned out to be. More a damsel in distress. He felt a hot surge of the old shame and self-loathing when he thought about all he had put Kim through. So far his cross-dressing had cost him his marriage and his family, and he was still confused about it. Years ago when it all came out in their therapy, it seemed like he and Kim would be able to work with these needs of his together. But they grew beyond what she could handle. Originally he had understood his intense need to cross-dress as being a psychological expression of his grief and yearning about the death of his mother. However, Dr. Karen Lawrence, the gender specialist, had suggested that there likely was more of a biological predisposition toward this behavior. Bob wasn't sure whether he agreed with her, but it certainly seemed to be the commonly held belief among the transgendered people he had gotten to know.

Now he was spending more and more time out and about in the world as Emily. He regularly attended his support group and saw his therapist in his feminine persona. He had gone to Saks Fifth Avenue once or twice and tried on clothes right along with the other women.

In their last therapy session three years ago, he had tried to explain to Kim that he wasn't ever going to be crazy enough to have an operation, but he still felt so much more in touch with his feelings when he was dressing in women's clothes.

"Expressing myself this way," and he paused and gestured toward his filled-out silk blouse and flowing skirt, "well, it just gives me some kind of glow of well-being." He looked down at the floor and sighed. "I know it doesn't make any sense. But it feels like, well, like I'm finally able to be the 'me' that I was always meant to be. I'm closer to the loving, gentle side of me."

Kim shook her head and looked away from him. "But Bob, I don't know why you think wearing these clothes makes you more loving. When you look like this, I feel like I'm with a complete stranger. Where's the man I married?"

"I'm still here and I still love you. Please try and hang in there with me. I had no idea things would turn out this way. I'm so sorry." Bob began to cry. "I know it's hard for you." He reached for her hand, but she recoiled from the touch of his painted nails.

Kim stood up and turned her back to him. Finally she whispered, "I don't think I can do this anymore. I still love you, but I don't know how to be married to this new you."

It was only six months after the divorce that she was diagnosed with breast cancer. It had already spread to the nodes. Right from the beginning they suspected that the radical mastectomy and the chemo wouldn't do it. Neither of them mentioned the similarity to his mother's cancer.

Gradually she let him help. He took over the shopping and the housecleaning as well as droving her to all the chemo treatments. They even shopped for a wig together.

"I suppose I should have gotten your advice on breast forms, too," she cracked, and they laughed. It was the first time after the divorce they'd joked about his other self.

Bob lay the roses down in the back seat. He hoped that Sarah and Bobby wouldn't think his idea of their each tossing one onto the grave was hopelessly sentimental. He wanted to wait until everyone else had gone and they would just be family again.

Bob could imagine the scene at the grave: him standing between Sarah and Bobby facing the dark hole with the fresh pile of soil next to it, watching the casket being lowered down into it. He visualized Kim lying in it, her wasted body and shrunken face.

Suddenly, the gesture with the roses seemed utterly stupid. He had to get through the day and be there for his kids as best he could. Hard enough. A surge of shame flooded him when he thought of Sarah's coolness since the divorce. He knew she knew, but they had never talked about it. She probably is disgusted and blames me for everything, he thought, the separation, wrecking the family. I'll have to talk with her. But not today. Today's for Kim. Bob's chest tightened and his eyes stung with tears.

He backed his Camry out of the driveway.

Just as Sarah was putting in her mother's diamond stud earrings, she heard the toot of her Dad's horn.

"Be there in a sec," she shouted down the stairs, even though she knew he couldn't hear her. She glanced at her watch. Exactly 11:45. God, he's punctual, she thought. He always came to the hospital right on the dot of 3 P.M. when the other visitors were allowed.

She hadn't had much to say to him throughout her mom's illness. He seemed in so many ways just like her old Dad. She tried not to think about his new identity issues. She hadn't told a soul. In her heart she felt like she had lost both parents.

"He's still your dad," her mom gently reminded her.

It annoyed Sarah how much her mother looked forward to his visits, calling them the "high point of my day." Sarah had sat dutifully on the right side of the bed while her mom turned toward him on the other side. At some point he'd bring out his "goodies" bag and pull out a little funny card, or some forbidden sweets, and always a cutout of "Arlo and Janis," Mom's favorite comic strip. He'd often shyly offer Sarah a Caramello bar, one of her childhood favorites.

In the last weeks, he read out loud to her mother from one of Mom's special childhood books, *Black Beauty*. The scene was so sweet it made Sarah uncomfortable. She had never seen her dad be that attentive and gentle before. He was being tenderly nurturing just like a—oh, for god sake—she realized he was acting just like a woman. Her dad was being caring like her mom would have been if the roles had been reversed. I didn't just lose a mother, I'm getting a new one. We're definitely not in Kansas anymore, Toto, she thought, smiling in spite of herself.

"Oh, well," she muttered as she glanced at the finished product in the mirror. Just as she turned to go downstairs, the car horn sounded again.

The dazzling bright day hit her as she stepped out the front door. There was her dad standing by the car in his blue serge suit. She hurried toward him.

They hugged.

"Oh, Daddy."

As she slid into the front seat beside him, she noticed his hands gripping the wheel. He was staring forward. He looked so lost and so sad.

"That's her dress, isn't it?" he said softly.

"Yes, she'd be amazed I could get in it."

Bob turned toward her and his eyes were wet with tears. "You know you kind of look like her in it, sweetie. You look so grown-up."

"You know what, Daddy?"

"No what?"

"I think I am grown-up." She smiled, reached over, and gently patted his right hand.

QUESTIONS FOR DISCUSSION

1. Does what happened with Bob and Kim 14 years after "Lunar Missions" change your feelings about what happened between them in the first story? Was Bob's becoming so deeply involved with transgendered behavior inevitable? How do you feel about him now?

2. It isn't clear from either story whether Bob's cross-dressing is more nature or nurture. What do you think? Is there a destiny that most people have, or are events in life mostly discontinuous and unpredictable?

3. Sarah is feeling the loss of both parents, but by the end she seems to have made a shift. What is it? How do you feel about it?

4. How do you feel about people with different sexual orientations or gender identity issues? How might you feel if this person were your spouse or child?
5. What makes it difficult to treat people who are of a different race, gender, sexual orientation, or ethnic background? How do you overcome these difficulties?

HEART TO HEART

"You know it's not just therapy when you go in there wondering about your choice of underwear," Sally said with a brittle smile, and then she started to cry again. "Harold's never going to understand. He'll kill me. I'm just not ready to tell him." Sally kept twisting her thick gold wedding band as she talked.

"I know this is hard," Jack Evans replied. "But I feel you're really putting your marriage at risk by not letting him in on it."

"You don't know my husband. I'm just frightened of him. I wish you could explain it to him. I'm sure he would listen to you."

Sally looked at Jack for reassurance. She was sitting on her hands, her knees were pressed together, and her feet were turned to- ward each other so the tips of her shoes were touching. She looked like a frightened schoolgirl.

"Maybe he can come in for a session after you tell him. We'll help Harold understand what happened. Fran Cohen has a colleague who runs a group for spouses of victims. That might be helpful."

"I can't imagine Harold doing that. But I'll make myself tell him. I really will. Promise. But, you know, Harold is actually the least of my worries. I don't feel ready for any of this. It's all going too fast."

"What's going too fast?" Jack asked. But he knew perfectly well. Jack felt the process was already out of his hands. He had referred her to a group run by Fran Cohen, a social worker who specialized in working with women who have been abused by therapists. Jack felt the group had pushed her prematurely to prosecute. When he discussed it with Fran, she stated flatly that it was an absolutely necessary part of the healing process for the victim to confront the perpetrator. "You do think it's critical that people like Arnold be stripped of their license, don't you?"

"Of course I do," said Jack, but he wasn't so sure. Fran was a gifted clinician, but in recent years she had become intensely single-minded in her pursuit of sexually abusive therapists. Jack wondered whether she was putting her need to see justice done ahead of Sally.

Confronting the perpetrator might be healing for some women, but sometimes the legal process could be just as abusive as the original events. Jack didn't know what the Medical Licensing Board was like, but psychiatrists were not noted for policing themselves well, particularly in a case of his word against hers.

He looked at Sally, who seemed so lost and, frankly, innocent. She was still having a hard time even understanding Sam Arnold's behavior as abuse.

"Sally, you have to remember this isn't your fault, and just because I've said I'm willing to testify doesn't mean that you have to go through with it."

"It means so much to me, Dr. Evans, that you offered to testify." She smiled at him as if he were her knight in shining armor. "I wouldn't be able to do this without your help. I do want to do it. It's not that I'm a feminist or anything like that. I do believe it's the right thing to do. I'm just scared, that's all."

"You and the group have all said that I shouldn't think of this as an affair, but sometimes I don't know what to think." Sally stared down at her hands, and her voice dropped to a whisper. "I mean, I've already told you, the main reason I went to him was my problem, you know, about not being able to have an orgasm. Not that I really minded that much, but Harold made such a big deal about it. I had asked him to come with me, but he thinks "shrinks" are for the birds. Obviously, I should have gone to see a woman therapist, but I thought I would learn more about men from a man."

Sally hesitated. "I went there to work on sex right from the start. Can that be held against me, Dr. Evans?" Sally looked at him pleadingly, as if with the wave of a hand he might grant her absolution.

"I can't imagine it could be. But that would be a good question to ask Fran. I'm sorry that I don't know more about the technicalities of this, but, as you know, this is my first time through this sort of proceeding myself."

Sally burst into tears again. "I've heard they ask really specific questions, like what we did and how many times. God, it makes my skin crawl. And what am I going to do if he denies it all. My lawyer says he might claim that I'm acting out some kind of psychotic transference or that I have a 'borderline personality disorder.' I don't know what any of that means, but he says it can be worse than a rape case, because the typical defense is to claim the patient is insane. Do you think they'll believe me?"

"I'm sure they will, Sally. All you have to do is tell the truth." Jack tried to sound confident and convincing. He had his own doubts about whether Sally was ready to go before the Board, but the hearing was scheduled and he didn't want to undermine her with his doubts. She was right to be worried, and she hadn't even told her husband yet.

"And besides," she continued, "four of the five on the panel are men and they're all psychiatrists like Sam. So who are they going to believe? And how do I explain that this all started four years ago and that I kept going back of my own free will and . . . "

"Whoa there, Sally, slow down, now you're going a little fast. This isn't a witch hunt. But it is frightening. Of course you're scared. Remember, you don't have to do this unless it's right for you."

I know I don't want to go through this mess, Jack said to himself as he glanced at the clock on his desk. He was dreading the whole process. It looked as if his testimony might be critical. He didn't want to be cross-examined by the Board. It is the nature of therapy that much of what is done is open to challenge because there is so little agreement about methodology. Suppose they decided to challenge his work with Sally?

Jack also didn't want to confront the defendant, Sam Arnold, whom he personally liked. He hadn't talked with Sam in several years, but Sam had been an enthusiastic member of one of his supervision groups. Sam clearly cared deeply about his clients. Jack remembered Sam presenting the case of the suicidal woman he had hospitalized. After several alarming phone messages, he had gone to her house and pleaded with her for several hours until she consented to letting him drive her to the hospital. He was the kind of guy willing to go the extra mile, but did this kind of caring become overinvolvement and a lack of boundaries? Maybe the same codependent characteristics were part of what also led to his behavior with Sally.

Remembering Sam's case made Jack wince as he considered what he might have done differently to help him. He had known that Sam's personal life had been quite difficult. Sam had mentioned to the group that he and his wife were about to institutionalize their 10-year-old son. Timmy was severely retarded and they couldn't adequately care for him anymore. Sam choked up as he talked about it with the group. Jack wished he had pulled Sam aside and found out if he and his wife were getting help. His involvement with Sally must have started around the same time.

Still, Jack couldn't imagine how Sam let himself get into this nightmare. He wondered about his side of the story. Of course, he reminded himself that explanations are never an excuse. But what if he had reached out to Sam a little more back then?

But now Sally was Jack's main concern. How would she handle the pressure? Would her marriage survive this crisis? Should it? He felt uncomfortable pushing her so hard to tell Harold, but he felt deeply that avoiding that confrontation was undermining the chances that the marriage could be salvaged. He was undoubtedly going to find out sooner or later, and maybe not directly from her. That would really be a disaster. Sometimes you just have to go with your hunches.

Jack was tempted to talk her into postponing the case, but he wasn't sure about his motives. Whose interests was he protecting? He felt cowardly and ambivalent at the same moment he was trying to project confidence and commitment.

"Listen, Sally, there's no excuse for a therapist being sexual with his patients. It's basically the same as incest. Patients are too vulnerable and too dependent to be able to resist."

"I keep needing you to say that." Sally reached for the tissue. "I feel like it was me. Why did I keep going back? I even kept paying his fee, week after week. Toward the end, we didn't even talk about my problems. I would just walk in, he'd lock the door behind me, and we'd fall into each other's arms."

"People do blame themselves. I remember sitting with a woman whose father had abused her when she was seven years old, and she was sure that it was her fault because he'd only done it to her and not her sisters. She thought she was to blame because she used to like to sit in his lap for bedtime stories."

"Dr. Evans, I wasn't seven."

Jack was silenced. She was right. She wasn't seven.

"I know, Sally." He hesitated, trying to find the right words. "I'm not sure anything I can say will really help right now. But in a therapy relationship, you're supposed to be able to trust the therapist totally so that you can risk exposing yourself. That's how it works. You do become almost as powerless as a child. Naturally, you want the love and approval of your therapist, just like all of us want it from our own parents. If the therapist uses that yearning to consummate his own sexual needs, that's criminal."

Jack wasn't connecting with her. It sounded more like he was hiding behind his therapist role—more talking at her, not with her.

"Dr. Evans, I know you want me to see myself as an innocent victim. I appreciate that." Sally paused. Her face was mottled and her eyes puffy. She looked him straight in the eye for the first time in the meeting. "But you don't get it."

Her voice rose. "I went to his office for a year after it started. We made love every Thursday at three o'clock. I looked forward to it. I had an orgasm every time. It was the best sex I ever had. I liked it. No, I loved it!" Sally almost shouted, and then she began to moan. "And what's worse, I loved him. I really did."

Jack sat back in his chair. Sally's outburst surprised him. Gone was the "little girl" routine. She sounded like a strong woman, trying to take responsibility for her own adult actions.

"It's okay, Sally," Jack said. He moved his chair closer to her. "Going through this is all part of it. Just let it happen. This takes time. It takes a long time."

Jack sat still while Sally wept. He knew she had to go through this pain and there were no words to soften it. He just leaned forward.

After a while, she blew her nose, grabbed more tissues, and wiped her eyes. She gave him a slight smile. "I must look like a mess."

"Not to worry," he said lightly, though he was still very worried himself. He still hadn't found a way of helping her get beyond heaping all the blame on herself. He decided to switch tacks.

"By the way, Sally, we're almost out of time, but I have a question for you. You're daughter's named Cynthia, right? How old is she?"

"She's 14."

"Can you imagine her being a grown woman?"

"Sure, she seems pretty grown-up already. What are you getting at?"

"Well, think about her for a second. Suppose 15 years from now Cynthia went into therapy because she felt terrible about herself. Her marriage was in trouble and she felt the problems were all her fault. Suppose instead of helping her, the therapist took advantage of her desperate need for reassurance and started an affair with her. Would you blame her for that?"

Sally sat up straighter on the sofa. Her jaw hardened. "Of course not. I'd be furious."

Then she suddenly smiled, "Okay, Doc, you made your point."

"Well, try to remember it, will you?"

*   *   *

Sam Arnold tilted back in his leather chair with his feet up on his desk and looked around his office as if he were seeing it for the last time. It was decorated in a colorful pastiche of Native American rugs, wall hangings, and big comfortable stuffed chairs. Behind the brown sofa there was a large portrait of Sitting Bull. On the opposite wall there hung a colorful framed weaving that supposedly had belonged to a Navajo medicine man. On top of his bookcase he had a collection of Indian peace pipes that he had collected on Martha's and his annual trip to the Southwest. The only obvious exception to the Native American theme was an abstract silver sculpture on a chrome and glass coffee table in front of the sofa. The sculpture was heavy and full in the base and seemed to flow upward to rounded and asymmetrical points. Some of his clients thought it was flickering fire. Others described it as a silver tulip. One female medical student saw it as an ovary about to release an egg.

Sam was a big, balding man. He had just turned 40. His wife, Martha, had pulled off a surprise square dance with a caller and band for his birthday. Although Sam was considerably overweight, with a big, lumbering bearish body, he was a square dancing enthusiast. He and Martha were cofounders of a square dancing group called the Square Pegs Society. Sam couldn't help wondering what would happen to the group once the word was out about him. He shook his head. It was a little premature to think about the group's response when he hadn't even figured out what to tell Martha.

It was easier for Sam to think about the square dancing group than to pick up the phone and call his lawyer. He wasn't ready to find out the date of the hearing. Once the date was known and duly marked down in the appointments book, just as if it were a client hour, then there was no longer any hope of escape. Each day, each hour shoved him toward it. Up to this point, Sam had fended off his anxiety with fantasies about the charges being dropped and Sally forgiving him. He even considered just disappearing. One day he called the Bureau of Indian Affairs to see if there was a need for psychiatrists in the Health Service. He suspected they might take anyone, even a psychiatrist with a ruined reputation and a suspended license.

Instead of calling Beasley, Sam twiddled over his alternatives. He still hadn't decided whether to acknowledge everything and throw himself on the mercy of the Board or to try to stonewall his way through it with a "her word against mine" defense. Protecting himself by denying Sally seemed truly criminal, but his lawyer had told him it was a sure bet. Beasley had said in their meeting, with a harsh chuckle, "We call it 'The Woman Scorned Defense.' " We just say that you properly rejected her inappropriate advances and now she's trying to punish you."

Sam sighed heavily. He couldn't be such a shit to Sally. He was still in love with her.

The therapy had been rewarding right from the beginning. At the end of the first meeting, she got up to leave and said, "This feels like it will be really helpful." She paused, "What do I call you? Dr. Arnold?"

"No, most of my clients just call me Sam."

"Well then," she said with a bright smile, "Thank you, Sam."

By the third session, Sally was making her first tentative steps to opening up. She was terribly shy about talking about sexual issues. Actually, he was too. Talking about sex had never been his forte. He probably should have referred her to a woman or a sex therapist right then. He had never treated a woman for specifically sexual issues before. But she seemed so earnest, eager, and trusting. She said she wanted him to help her understand men better.

"My husband wants to do it almost every day! I can't imagine it. Is that typical?"

"No, Sally, men have a wide variety of sexual needs, just like women. Most couples have to learn how to negotiate their different sexual drives."

"But, I don't know what I want. I don't think I've ever—you know." She glanced out the window, took a deep breath, and pressed on: "You know, had an orgasm. At least I don't think I have. But I'm not sure. It's always over so quickly anyway. I know that sounds dumb, and I've read that women are always complaining about its going too fast. But it does go too fast for me. Is there any way that I can encourage him to go more slowly? Harold gets very offended if I try to talk with him about this. He says that it's my problem, and that's why I need a shrink."

Sam smiled and reached for his pipe. "Well, Sally, when it comes to creating problems in the bedroom, it usually takes two to not tango."

Sally actually laughed out loud. She was clearly relieved.

Sam was quite taken with her full, deep laughter. She seemed very appreciative.

In the sessions that followed they made rapid progress. He introduced Sally to the Nancy Friday books on women's sexual fantasies and encouraged her to explore masturbation. He encouraged her to keep a journal of her sexual feelings, which she called her "Purple Passion" book. They role played her learning how to talk with Harold about her needs as well as how to say no comfortably to him. Sometimes Sam would play Harold's role. Other times he would play Sally and she would demonstrate how Harold usually responded.

Sally blossomed right before his eyes. She was still not orgasmic with her husband, but she was much more comfortable with her own sexuality and had even ventured out and bought a vibrator.

"Right after our last session," she had reported with a triumphant smile. "I hid it in the back of my lingerie drawer. Harold would be shocked."

Sam was a faithful husband and had never even considered crossing the line with a client. He was confident that he wouldn't with Sally. He cared too much about her. But he could feel his attraction grow. He liked her simple elegance. She wore long flowing skirts with ivory silk blouses. He liked her soft brown hair that fell to her shoulders and her long dangling earrings, especially the silver Indian feather ones. She wore silver and turquoise necklaces and belts that seemed to just blend into his office motif. Like she belonged there.

It shocked him the first time he caught himself imagining making love to Sally in the middle of his regular Saturday night session with his wife. She would never be adventuresome enough to go out and buy a vibrator. Martha was an eyes-closed, lights-out, missionary position kind of wife. Sam tried to stimulate a little variety in their sex life by giving her some of the Nancy Friday books, but as far as he could tell, she had never taken a peek at them. After they had to put Timmy in Green Hills, Martha had just given up on even pretending to care about sex. Their Saturday nights were painfully perfunctory. Sam tried to be as gentle and as understanding as possible, but he still felt he was just an annoyance.

In his work with Sally, Sam began to use his own experiences to teach her about men. He convinced himself that it would help her to not idealize him. Perhaps it would even make her more accepting of her husband's limitations.

"You know, Sally, speaking as a man here, I think I can understand how your husband feels. All of us grow up feeling like we're responsible for pleasing women. Men have a big ego investment in being good lovers. And we have a lot of anxiety no matter how confident we appear to be."

"I'm sure your wife appreciates how open and honest you are. Not many men are able to talk about these things."

"Well, I have my flaws like any other man. Certainly my wife could tell you that. But, getting back to your husband, I suspect he feels like you're disappointed in him."

"I wouldn't be if he would just talk to me. That's more important than sex. It's so easy to talk to you. I never thought I could be this open with a man. I feel so lonely sometimes with Harold. When he's done, he just turns his back and goes to sleep. It's like I don't matter to him at all. It's awful. I'm left lying there with his stuff dripping out of me."

Then Sally began to cry hard. "I just feel like a used tissue."

Sam moved his chair next to her and took her hand. "You need to be appreciated for who you are. You're a very special lady, Sally Bainbridge, and don't you forget it."

Sally squeezed his hand and looked him in the eyes with deep gratitude.

At the end of that session, Sally asked shyly if she could have a hug. It seemed natural and appropriate given how intense the session had been and how needy Sally seemed to be. But when Sam embraced her, he noticed that he had to lean forward from the waist so that she wouldn't inadvertently press against his erection.

Somehow, in the sessions that followed, the end-of-the-meeting hugs became full body embraces. He couldn't remember who initiated them. It seemed mutual. Making love became inevitable.

It was wonderful.

Sam smacked his desk with his fist. Thinking like this just made it worse. He was horrified by what he had done. How he could he have been so stupid? Not only had he probably destroyed his career, he had also potentially wrecked Sally's life. He felt like such a shit.

His hand picked up the phone and dialed Beasley's number. The hearing date would be January 15th, the same day his quarterly taxes were due.

*   *   *

Sally sat in her car with both hands on the wheel. She was in the parking lot next to the soccer field where Cynthia's team was practicing. Although she rarely came to watch Cynthia play, she couldn't stand sitting in the house anymore waiting for Harold. Surprising Cyn with a girl's night out invitation seemed like an excellent plan.

Sally watched Cyn challenge another girl for the ball. She was so tall and lithe, she could be a ballerina, but she played soccer like she was a linebacker. Sally couldn't really see Cyn being dumb enough and weak enough to let herself get caught in a situation like hers. Cyn was much more independent and assertive than Sally had been when she was a teenager. Not a wimp like her mother: She's tough, more like Harold.

Sally remembered the white-water canoe trip she had taken with Harold shortly after they first started going out. She was nauseated with fear: afraid of the water ever since childhood. But she feigned enthusiasm for his carefully planned trip down the Kennebec River in Maine. Harold had made it clear that being outdoorsy was a necessary ingredient in a future Mrs. Bainbridge and Sally had already set her sights on being the one to fill that role. She borrowed the appropriate outfit from her roommate, took a Dramamine just in case, and greeted Harold with an enthusiastic grin at 6:00 that Saturday morning.

On the car ride up, Harold regaled Sally with his vast knowledge of white-water technique. When he asked her about her experience on rivers, she managed to parlay her one Girl Scout canoeing trip across a placid pond into sounding like a major adventure. She didn't share that even that trip had been scary for her.

Slowly, over the course of that endless day, Sally could feel her perky Girl Scout smile deteriorate into a frozen grimace. Fortunately Harold never noticed. She was in the bow of the canoe and he was preoccupied with his various steering maneuvers. He barked out orders from the stern about which side of the canoe to paddle on. She would take furtive stabs at the water. The canoe paddle felt as foreign as a baseball bat. The rocks seemed to come hurtling toward her out of the surging water. There was a steady roar of noise. She was soaked to the skin. Her hair was wet, stringy, and stuck to her face like overcooked spaghetti. She regretted that she had bothered to get up at 4:30 to wash and set it.

Her session with the Board and the confrontation with Harold were rushing at her just like the rocks on the Kennebec. She was being swept along. Evans, Cohen, the group, and her lawyer were all telling her what to do. It made her feel even more helplessly out of control.

Sally was unsure which she dreaded most: giving her deposition to the Board or telling Harold. He wasn't going to take it well. Dr. Evans had advised her to bring Harold in for a session. Fat chance. Harold believed in a "pull yourself up by the bootstraps" approach to life that didn't leave much room for therapists. The very thought of how he would respond to her story about Sam Arnold made her shudder.

Sally caught herself wishing that she could call Sam, just to hear his gentle, comforting voice. It had been over a year since they had talked, but she still missed him. She didn't know love could feel the way it did with him. Her whole week revolved around what they called "our time." She gave up drinking, lost 10 pounds, and was even much sweeter to Harold. It was a delicious time.

Then she wrecked it. She told Sam that she was going to leave Harold and take an apartment near his office, and was completely blindsided by the horror-stricken look on his face.

"But, Sally, you can't turn your life upside down for us. I can't even consider leaving Martha. Not after everything she's been through. I'm so sorry."

He reached for her but she slipped away from his embrace and ran out of his office. He called her and begged her to come back, but everything had changed. The next session he told her that he had made a terrible mistake with her and that he couldn't allow her to put her life in jeopardy. Finally, he said that they had to stop meeting for her sake, no matter how desperately hard it might be for him.

The last time, they held each other and cried for almost the whole hour. It was the right thing to do, but she couldn't imagine living without him: his gentleness and acceptance. She could still feel the transcendent moment of their first embrace. How tender it was, how safe she felt.

She never should have told Evans or even gone to see him. It was Sam's last suggestion. "I trust him," Sam had said.

But telling Evans was what set this whole mess in motion. He sent her to that Cohen woman and . . .

"Mom, what are you doing here?" Cynthia yelled through the closed window.

Sally rolled down the window. "Hi, honey. I just wanted to see how you're doing. I thought we might have a bite at Papa Gino's and hit the mall."

"Oh, Mom, don't you remember? I'm supposed to go over to Mary's house to work on our term paper. Her mother's picking us up any minute."

Sally smiled, hiding her disappointment. "That's right. I forgot. You run along then. I'll see you at home later."

Sally watched enviously as Cynthia ran over to Mary and a gaggle of girls. What she would give to be one of them fretting over term papers, cute boys, and soccer scores.

She started the car. Somehow she'd tell Harold before they went to bed that night.

After she finished the dishes, Sally found Harold holed up in his office in front of his computer, and plunged awkwardly into the topic.

"I've got some very upsetting things I have to talk to you about. Please let me just blurt it all out without interrupting me, okay?"

Harold glowered throughout her description of the events with Arnold.

"He kept encouraging me to be more and more open about my sexuality. And I figured that I needed to do that because you were always complaining about how uptight I was. One session he massaged my neck to help me release tension. I wanted so badly for it to work between you and I. It seemed supportive and appropriate when he started hugging me at the end of sessions. He said he hugged all of his clients. Then he started talking about himself and his marriage. Before too long, the hugs became more insistent, but I didn't know what to say or what was happening.

Sally was appalled at how self-serving her story sounded, but she couldn't stop. "Anyway, I didn't know if I was just being uptight about it all. Dr. Evans says it's normal for clients to be unable to resist when these situations start happening."

Harold was clenching his fists and on the verge of exploding. She continued, "Evans says that victims are just so ashamed that they can't tell anyone, least of all their husbands and. . . . "

"As well they should be goddamn ashamed," Harold cut in. His face was red and contorted. "You fucked this shrink of yours for over a year, and you're claiming this was abuse! What is this bullshit! You pay a fucking shrink every week out of my checkbook and you want me to believe that you're a victim? This new idiot, what's-his-name, Evans, says it's like incest. It's the biggest pile of manure I ever heard of!"

Harold was out of his seat and standing over her raging, "You used to come home and tell me what a wonderful man Arnold was. How he made you feel so much better about yourself. I don't believe this. I want you out of here!"

"Please Harold, I'm sorry. Don't shout. Cynthia will be home any minute. Please, you don't understand. It wasn't like you think."

"Oh, really," Harold said in a low, cold voice. "Am I talking quietly enough for you? After all, we wouldn't want Cynthia to come in and find out that her mother bought sex from her psychiatrist. I'm sure your daughter would be impressed."

Sally buried her face in her hands and whispered, "I'm so sorry, I'm so sorry."

"Sorry, my ass!"

Sally looked up at him with tears streaming down her face. "Please just come with me one time to Dr. Evans's. He can explain this to. . . . "

"So I can pay him to tell me that my wife is just a poor innocent victim? Get real. I don't want anything to do with any of those assholes!"

Then Harold turned his back to her. There was a moment of silence. Then in an even tone, he said, "Get the fuck out of here."

*   *   *

Jack Evans stared at the computer screen. The title of his article, "Heart to Heart: New Pathways to Intimacy," loomed over the blank page. Jack was tired and annoyed. Intimacy was the farthest thing from his mind. He was preoccupied with this business about Sally and the Board and feeling a little guilty about leaving Ellen with the kids' homework duties.

He felt torn about Sally. In a way, it was good for her to take some responsibility for her behavior in the relationship with Arnold. She was right. She wasn't seven. Accepting the consequences of her own actions actually seemed like a step forward for her. On the other hand, he genuinely believed that she had been criminally abused. She should no more be blaming herself than a rape victim should be blamed for not resisting aggressively enough or for wearing a short skirt.

But he had an uneasy feeling that having been manipulated by Arnold, Sally was now being manipulated by Fran, the group, and himself. His job was to help Sally find her own voice.

He wondered if he was going to have to testify in front of Sam. The poor bastard had really screwed up. He had taken advantage of Sally and frankly deserved to get burned. Yet Jack hated to see anyone go through the humiliation that Sam would have to face. What if . . .

The phone rang. Jack didn't pick it up.

Ellen called upstairs. "Jack, the phone. It's for you."

"Shit," muttered Jack out loud as he reached for the extension.

"Oh, Dr. Evans, this is Sally. I'm so glad to be able to reach you. I'm sorry to bother you at home, but I just had to talk with you. My husband is furious. I tried to tell him what you've explained to me and I just couldn't get through to him. He's threatening divorce."

"Did you suggest to him that the three of us meet?"

"I did, but he said no. I don't know. . . . I'm so confused. Tell me what should I do."

Dammit, Jack thought, he should have prepared her better for this. "Give him some time to come around, Sally. You've been wrestling with this horrible mess for a while now. He's only just found out. It's going to take time for the shock to wear off. Just hang in there and I'll see you on Thursday. And you know that if you need to, you can call again."

"Thank you, Dr. Evans, I don't know what I would do without you. I couldn't get through this alone."

"Okay, Sally, take care."

As he hung up the phone, Jack felt a sour taste of irritation. Something about her breathy desperation annoyed him. He hoped she couldn't pick it up in his tone of voice. Besides, it was completely appropriate for her to be leaning on him during this crisis. Still, her slightly seductive, little-girl quality made him acutely uncomfortable. "Oh, Dr. Evans, I couldn't be doing this without you." Careful, Jack, he chided himself. Let's not get into blaming the victim here.

He clicked off the computer and headed downstairs to the TV room. The hell with the article.

*   *   *

Jack decided to call first thing in the morning before he had a chance to change his mind.

"Hi, Sam, this is Jack Evans."

There was a long pause.

Although they weren't friends or colleagues, Jack felt Sam deserved to know that he was going to testify, even though he was sure that Ms. Enright, Sally's lawyer, wouldn't have approved. Besides, Sam had referred Sally. Sam must have assumed that Jack would collude in keeping the situation under wraps in some way.

"Hello, Dr. Evans," said Sam softly.

"This is really awkward, Sam. I'm calling about the Board hearings coming up next week."

"I figured that." His voice was lifeless.

"I guess you know that I've been treating Sally Bainbridge, and I will be testifying in front of the Board."

"I've been informed to that effect."

"Well, listen, I wanted to tell you personally, because of our having worked together. I feel very bad about the whole situation. I don't know how this mess really occurred, but any one of us in this business is capable of making serious mistakes. We're all human. I'm very sorry, but I do have to go through with this."

Another long pause. What was he saying? Jack wondered, hearing himself almost apologizing to Sam. He felt excruciatingly stupid to have made the call.

"This call might not even be appropriate, Sam. I just wanted to let you know personally. The other thing is that I honestly hope you'll be able to acknowledge what happened. There's treatment for this kind of thing, and. . . . "

"I don't think I should be having this conversation with you, Dr. Evans. My lawyer has advised me not to discuss the particulars of these charges with anyone."

After the phone call, Jack stared out the window of his office. He looked at his lawn littered with the red and gold of dead leaves. The weekend of raking seemed like a vast improvement over this situation. He knew he was doing the right thing, but he felt like a snitch. Maybe he should have contacted Sam much earlier and encouraged a meeting between him and Sally. Perhaps this could have been resolvable in a less destructive manner. After all, Sam wasn't an evil predator.

On the other hand, the guy should have kept it buttoned.

*　　*　　*

It was 10:10 A.M.. All but two of the Board members had arrived. They sat behind a long mahogany table. Dr. Jerome Leavit, head of the New England Psychoanalytic Institute, was chatting amiably with his protégé, Dr. James Goodwin. Dr. Frank Gutcheon was leafing through the sports pages. The lone woman on the Board, Dr. Harriet Denby, sat off by herself and was making notes. So far none of them had looked directly at Jack.

To Jack's right at a small desk was a stenographer; Sally was to his left. She was conservatively dressed in a black wool suit. She sat demurely with her ankles crossed and her hands folded in front of her. She was sitting between her husband, Harold, and her lawyer, Judy Enright. Harold Bainbridge was a small, wiry man with slicked-back black hair and wire-rimmed glasses. He had on a three-piece suit. Their heads were bent toward each other as he and the lawyer whispered together.

Jack looked out the big picture window at the Boston skyline. In the distance, he could see the crew sculls plowing along the Charles. They looked as delicate as water bugs. Then he glimpsed over at Harold, and remembered his only meeting with the guy. Jack had opened the session with a self-deprecating joke about shrinks, but Harold didn't betray even a hint of a smile. Instead he launched in about how grossly Sally had betrayed him. Finally, after making no headway explaining how these things can happen, Jack declared, "Mr. Bainbridge, you know, it wasn't just Sally who was abused by Dr. Arnold. You and your marriage have also been profoundly harmed by his unethical behavior. That's why you have every right to sue him yourself."

Harold latched onto this idea and began firing questions at Jack about the legal process. Jack instantly regretted mentioning them pursuing their own suit. It wasn't meant as a literal suggestion so

89

much as a way of being supportive. It turned out to be throwing chum to a shark.

Jack recommended a support group for spouses, but Harold replied, "I'm not going to sit around with a bunch of hand-wringing whiners. We'll take care of this matter in court."

Jack looked around the hearing room. This was supposed to be only an informal hearing, but the scene in the room looked like a set for a TV courtroom melodrama.

At least Sam Arnold wasn't there. Jack didn't want to face him. Knowing that his testimony would have a strong impact on the Board's deliberations, it would have been difficult to administer the *coup de grâce* in front of Sam.

*　　*　　*

The Chairman of the Board called the meeting to order. Sally spoke almost in a whisper. She had rehearsed her presentation with Judy and Fran, but she was still nervous. She also felt guilty about the way her reconstruction of events had become more one-sided. Judy had told her that it was necessary for her to present the matter in a pretty black-and-white way because of the Board's potential bias in favor of Arnold, but Sally was worried about being fair.

"Then he began offering to massage the tension out of my neck. He said he had learned this in his bioenergetics training. It was about that time that he suggested we hug at the end of the sessions. I was unsure about this, but he reassured me that it was perfectly normal."

Sally paused and reached into her purse for a handkerchief, just in case. Sally wished she hadn't lied about that first hug, but having told Harold that Sam had initiated the hugs, now she was stuck with it. She reminded herself that the rest of the story was basically true and that regardless of how the hugs started, Evans had reassured her there was still no excuse for Arnold to take advantage of her.

"In the next session when it really started, we were role playing," Sally continued. "He said he wanted to teach me how to give 'encouraging feedback' (that's what he called it), so that I could communicate better with Harold. We sat on the sofa. He pretended that he was Harold and was making overtures, and I was to tell him how I wanted to be touched and then he started touching me. . . . "

Sally began to cry. "Do I have to tell every detail of this?"

Dr. Leavit emptied his pipe in the ashtray. "No, Mrs. Bainbridge, we just need to know when the actual sexual acts began and the length of time you and Dr. Arnold continued to have relations."

"You mean, how long did it last? It was only a 50-minute hour."

The solemnity of the occasion imperceptibly cracked. Some of the Board members swallowed a smile. "No, Mrs. Bainbridge, I'm just asking approximately how many times you and Dr. Arnold had relations."

"I'd like to object." Judy Enright stood up. "The use of the phrase 'had relations' implies a consensual involvement. My client was truly under the sway of Dr. Arnold, and was literally unable to say no to him. This is not the same as 'having relations' with him."

"Your objection is duly noted, Ms. Enright. But this isn't a court-room. We're all just doing the best we can. As you know, it's quite difficult to find the right language to describe these sorts of events."

After Sally finished her story, members of the Board were free to ask questions.

Dr. Denby was the toughest questioner.

"Tell us, Mrs. Bainbridge, after Dr. Arnold began this sexual abuse, who did you tell?"

"I didn't tell anybody."

"And how long did you say this abuse happened?"

"As I said, I think it was almost a full year, but I'm not sure."

"And after it was over, who did you tell?"

"I didn't tell anyone until I told Dr. Evans."

"And that was how long after you stopped seeing Dr. Arnold?"

"Six months."

"How long after seeing Dr. Evans was it before you told your husband?"

"About a year."

"Just a minute," Enright jumped in. "It sounds like you're sug-gesting that my client's difficulty in acknowledging this abuse to anyone implies some culpability on her part."

"No, Ms. Enright, I'm just aware that apparently your client terminated the therapy without ever complaining to Dr. Arnold. She says she never confided in a friend or a relative. And if I heard her correctly, she only recently told her husband. I'm just trying to understand the process that's unfolded here, that's all." Dr. Denby folded her hands in front of her primly and smiled.

*   *   *

During the break, Jack headed for the men's room. He was confused. He thought that Sally had initiated the first hug. Not that it really made a difference but. . . . Then Harold stood beside him at the next urinal.

"Except for maybe that lady shrink, I think we got them all," he said, facing the wall in front of them both. "Sally was great. And you're going to be the icing on the cake, Doc. I can just feel it."

Jack zipped up and smiled wanly back at him. Clearly he smelled blood in the water.

Jack's testimony went next. When he began to explain the effects of therapist abuse, Dr. Denby interrupted him and said, "Dr. Evans, the Board appreciates your willingness to educate us on the nature of therapist abuse, but we feel adequately knowledgeable on this topic, and if you would simply confine your remarks to the specific discussion of Mrs. Bainbridge's case."

"Yes, Doctor."

"Mrs. Bainbridge came to you because she was still upset about her therapy with Dr. Arnold, is that right?"

"Yes, that's true."

"You've said that you learned about the sexual abuse within the first few sessions. And yet, as I understand it, the Board was not notified about these serious charges for six months. Mrs. Bainbridge said in her testimony that it was Ms. Cohen who encouraged her to notify the Board, not yourself. Would you favor us with your thinking on this issue, Dr. Evans?"

"Well, I felt strongly," Jack squirmed in his chair, "that my first responsibility was to Sal—I mean, Mrs. Bainbridge. I wanted to make sure she was ready to go through this painful process without incurring further damage."

"So you took it upon yourself to decide for Mrs. Bainbridge when she'd be able to handle reporting this? Do you feel that you had a responsibility to report this immediately yourself?"

"Look, Dr. Denby, it's my job to take care of my clients the best way I know how." Jack's voice began to rise. "I don't mean to sound defensive here, but I feel like I moved as quickly as was appropriate for my client. I'm sorry if you don't think so."

"Now, Dr. Evans, nobody is suggesting an error on your part," chimed in Dr. Leavitt with a smile. "We're just trying to understand your thinking about the case."

Jack stumbled through the rest of his testimony.

*   *   *

Sam was hoping to slip out of the house without seeing Martha, but she came into their bedroom while he was knotting his tie.

"Sam, why are you wearing a suit?" she asked.

"I have that review meeting this afternoon with the licensing Board about the complaint I told you about."

"You mean the woman who's accusing you of making sexual overtures because you decided to refer her to a mental hospital?"

"That's the one. I'm pretty sure this will be a formality. It's her word against mine and she's obviously psychotic."

"You don't seem very worried."

"It's just one of the risks of the trade." Sam smiled at Martha. "Wish me luck," he said.

"Are you going to be back in time for dinner tonight?"

"I don't think so. I don't know when I'll be home."

Sam almost vomited up his lunch on the way downtown. His thoughts raced in his head as he drove blindly along. He couldn't see any way out. He kept going over and over it. How did it happen? How could he have been so stupid?

Then the memory of holding Sally came back to him. Whatever anyone thought, he loved Sally. It had been so hard to break it off

with her, and since the whole process had started he had been thinking of her more and more often. He knew she'd testified this morning and he almost wished he could have been there just to see her.
He just wanted to talk with her. Tell her how sorry he was. He
yearned to take her in his arms one more time.

"Jesus, get a grip." He squeezed the steering wheel of his car.
The traffice slowed to a stop, and he surveyed the other drivers
around him, each in their own world. Here he was in his elegant for-
est green Saab. Certainly to the rest of his rush hour companions he
didn't look like he was going to his own funeral.

A couple of days ago, Sam had decided to tell the truth. At first
he felt relieved as he contemplated having his license revoked and
voluntarily offering to go into treatment for his problem. The current trend in the mental health field to accept many "acting-out"
behaviors as manifestations of a "disease" like sex addiction, worka-
holism, and the like would perhaps allow him to go through a purga-
tory period and then reemerge, hopefully with his family and profession intact.

I just have to get through the humiliation, he told himself.

He remembered being seven. He had just finished his bath and
was feeling lonely and bored as usual. He decided to try out his
father's razor. He lathered up carefully and then ran his thumb along
the razor's edge to see if there was a blade in there.

Blood spurted.

Panicking, Sam ran downstairs into the living room, calling for
his mother—"Mom, Mom, look." He held up his dripping thumb.

His mother was having one of her formal tea parties. All the ladies in the room turned and stared at the naked and chubby little
boy, his face covered in shaving cream. There was a moment of abso-
lute silence.

His Mother frowned, then flashed one of her best hostess smiles
and said, "Now Samuel, is this the way you've been taught to enter a
room?"

The ladies burst out laughing.

Mrs. Arnold, obviously pleased with herself, continued, "Do run along, put on some clothes and a Band-Aid. And, by all means, don't drip on the rug."

Sam ran out of the room to the sound of the ladies tittering. In his room later, he thought he would die.

His marriage to Martha, his professional success, and his expansive social life seemed to have carried him light years away from his lonely boyhood. Now his life seemed as fragile as one of his intricate Nauset Beach sand castles faced with a rising tide. In the next hour, it would all be swept away. He felt a wave of bitterness.

He looked at his watch. It was 1:30. The meeting was scheduled from 2:00 to 4:00. No matter what happened, it would be over in three hours. That thought gave him a tidbit of comfort.

Sam walked into the hearing feeling like that naked little boy. He sat down in front of them with Beasley next to him. In a slow monotone, he told his side of the story, tried to explain how inadvertently it had all begun and how sorry he was, and that he would do whatever was necessary to make amends.

The Board listened impassively.

Dr. Denby leaned forward and pulled her reading glasses down to the tip of her nose. "In your recollection, Dr. Arnold, did you initiate physical contact with your patient?"

Sam hesitated and then said, "Well, I certainly took her hand and held it when she was upset. I don't really remember how the rest of it got started." He wasn't about to start finger-pointing. "I just know this is all my fault."

"I suppose it wouldn't be in your notes . . . ?"

Dr. Leavit jumped in. "I don't think we need to go back over all the details, Dr. Denby. Dr. Arnold is accepting full responsibility, I believe."

"Yes, I am, Dr. Leavit," whispered Sam.

"Well, thank you, Dr. Arnold, for your candor. We will let you know the results of these deliberations as expeditiously as possible."

Dr. Denby sniffed and pursed her lips.

Sam just nodded.

*   *   *

Sally stirred her drink idly while she watched Harold pace back and forth in front of the phone in their kitchen. He had been trying to reach their lawyer all night, desperately wanting to find out how Dr. Arnold's part of the hearing had gone. She wished it were over. She hated Harold's blood lust and she hated herself for going along. She knew she was using it. The way she fawned over him as if he were a noble saviour, rescuing her from the savage rapist, disgusted her. But she felt she had no choice. She couldn't defend Sam. Harold would kill her.

She remembered the kindness in Sam's eyes, how they laughed together. She could almost hear his gentle and encouraging words. She remembered his touch. She wished they could talk just one more time.

*   *   *

Beasley had waited until the end of the hearing to inform Sam about the civil suit and that the Bainbridges weren't interested in negotiating. Any hope that he could get out of this was dashed.

"Mr. Bainbridge wants you tarred and feathered and run out of town on a rail. He's a real son of a bitch." Beasley had said.

Walking out of the building, Sam couldn't face going home. Thoughts of the stories in the paper, confessing it all to Martha and then his parents horrified him. He could imagine his mother's rage at him for embarrassing her. Undoubtedly they will lose the house and he will have to file for bankruptcy.

Sam spent a couple of hours sitting by the Esplanade as joggers, cyclists, and lovers holding hands swept by him. He felt like he'd just been told he had terminal cancer. The milling people around him felt miles away, as if he were looking at them through the wrong end of binoculars.

It was past 8:30 by the time Sam got home.

"Honey, is that you?" Martha called out from the kitchen.

"Yep, it's me."

"Come on in here. I saved you a bite to eat."

Sam walked into the kitchen. "I'm not hungry. I'm going to have a drink."

"Did the hearing go all right? You look dead tired."

"I think it will all be fine, but it was harder than I expected. Nowadays, any charges people want to sling are taken seriously. I couldn't believe it."

"Don't you think they'll be able to see that she's crazy?"

Sam looked at Martha with her pinched frown, the one she wore when they were talking about Timmy. "Don't worry, hon, I'm sure they will. But you can never tell about how the politics of it might work. But it will be okay. It's nothing to worry about."

"I'm going up to bed soon. Are you coming up?"

"Sure, I just have to make a few phone calls in my office."

Sam sat in his office. He stared at the portrait of Sitting Bull. The grim old warrior stared back at him. Then he went into his bathroom to get the bottle of Valium he had been using for his nerves the past few weeks. He had enough.

I should write a note, he thought, and took out a piece of his business stationery. He stared at the blank page and imagined Martha waking up in the middle of the night, noting the empty side of the bed, and padding down here in her slippers. He could see her terror, her frantic call to 911, and the sound of sirens roaring up their street. Maybe the ambulance would get there in time. Then what? Maybe he'd be brain-damaged like Timmy. The image of his poor sweet son with his crooked, goofy smile and his innocent wide eyes yanked at him.

He knew he couldn't do it. He crumpled up the page and threw it and the pills into his wastebasket. Was he just chickening out or was doing it more the coward's way out? He decided he would just have to go through whatever he had to go through.

He turned off the light, tilted back in his easy chair, and closed his eyes.

The phone rang.

"Sam?" whispered the voice on the other end of the line. "It's me, Sally."

"Oh, Sally," he sighed, and his face broke into a smile.

QUESTIONS FOR DISCUSSION

1. How did you feel about the way this case was being handled by Sam and Sally, by Jack Evans, by the Board? Were there any viable alternatives? Should Jack have tried to handle it privately between Sam and Sally?
2. How are your responses to Sam and Sally similar and/or different?
3. This is a story of therapist abuse. Is it also a love story?
4. What do you imagine happens with Sam and Sally after she calls him?
5. How do we assess the responsibility of both client and therapist when they have a consensual sexual relationship? Is it 100% the therapist's fault in all cases? Or are there mitigating circumstances in some instances?
6. Have you ever had romantic/erotic feelings as either a client or a therapist? Is that normal? What should either a client or a therapist do if they have these kinds of feelings in a therapeutic relationship?
7. How might your response to this story have felt different if the therapist had been a woman, either in a same-sex relationship or with a male client?

BLEEDING THE LINES

"Marvin spoils her to death. You have no idea. And Jennifer is just impossible. I swear the two of them drive me crazy." She glared at me. "It's unbelievable, Dr. Harney—all she has to do is click her fingers and she's off to the mall with oodles of cash." Joanna Crandall was off on a double-barreled rant.

I was literally sitting on my hands. These were the worst sessions: the ones where parents whine about their teenagers. I had started refusing referrals of families with teenagers, but I'd been seeing Joanna for years, so I had to see it through.

I leaned forward in my chair and nodded slightly at Joanna as if her every word was dripping with psychological significance. I stole a glance at the clock. Ten minutes to go. Come on, Beth. Hang in there, I said to myself

"Let me just show you the two of them together. They're like two peas in a pod." She reached into her purse and showed me a picture of her 16-year-old daughter with her father's arm draped around her shoulder. I felt a sharp pain rip through my body.

"Are you okay?" Joanna asked.

I really must have looked awful if she noticed. Usually I was prepared, but the picture hit hard. It wasn't Joanna's fault. She didn't know about Ally.

"I'm fine, Joanna, I just had a stitch in my side." I shifted in my chair. "Please go on. Your daughter may be a little bratty but she is very pretty too."

"Unfortunately she knows it. The boys are swarming like flies. Let me tell you another thing. . . . "

I barely breathed for the rest of the session. As she turned her back to leave, my smile hardened into a mask. I sat down at my desk, lay my head on my arms and closed my eyes, praying the tears would come. My eyes were as hard as marbles. The first year, I thought I would never stop crying, and now I couldn't cry at all. Crying is better.

Ally. Most of the time, my office was my sanctuary. I got lost in my clients' lives. Even in the first year, when my eyes glistened sometimes, most of my clients either didn't notice or seemed to feel more deeply cared about. Losing Ally made me both a better and worse therapist. I understood and connected to my clients' suffering much more deeply. On the other hand, when someone like Joanna was complaining about her child not getting 700s on her SATs, I would almost scream, "Be goddamn grateful that your kid's alive to take the stupid tests!"

Still I was better being Dr. Beth Harney than being Mrs. Peter Harney. With Peter, I was as missing in action as he was. I ate dinner by myself, usually a bowl of soup while standing at the kitchen counter staring at the headlines about a world I didn't belong in any more. On weekends, I rode in the woods on my horse, Sky. It was just about the only real relief I ever felt.

Peter worked late every night and on weekends he went into the office to write opinions. He finally became a judge and he was good at it. He looked the part in his black robes and his full head of silvery gray hair. But even serving on the bench, he was killing himself the way he did when he was in politics. He was hiding behind his work too.

The phone rang. Undoubtedly Peter, letting me know he'd be working late. I almost never heard from anyone else. People couldn't take being around us anymore. I didn't blame them. I didn't want to be around me either. And I didn't want to see them and hear how their kids were doing at Harvard or Podunk U. I picked up the phone.

"It's me."

"Quelle surprise," I said too tartly.

"Bad day?" he asked.

"No, just the usual."

"Well, looks like . . . "

"You're going to be late again," I cut him off.

"Come on, Beth."

"I'm sorry, Peter," I sighed and looked out the window, "I am in a foul mood and it's . . . "

"Listen, I've got to run. They're calling us back into chambers."

With Ally gone we didn't have much to talk about. She was the centerpiece of our lives—probably the main reason Peter came back after all. The couple therapy helped us patch our marriage back together, but I had a hard time letting myself fully go with Peter after his affair with Nancy. Christ, that woman cast a long shadow. Fourteen years. We never talked about it outside of therapy. We threw ourselves into raising Ally. I told myself we would work out the intimacy stuff later on, like other couples I knew.

So we worked hard and built a life on the foundation of Ally. Fortunately she was a delight to be with, and every weekend we adventured together: backpacking, skiing, tennis, and sailing. When Ally discovered sports with Peter she dropped her interest in girly things and changed into a powerhouse of fiery athletic energy.

And Peter was into it, too. As hard driving as Peter could be at work, when it came to time with Ally, he was equally creative and energetic. Peter had us welcome in each season with "The Harney Magical Mystery Tour." I got to tag along but I knew it was mostly for Ally.

In April 1994, just before Ally's 10th birthday, he actually packed Ally's and my suitcases secretly and told us to be in the car at 8 P.M. Friday night, no questions asked. I was shocked when he led us onto his rich friend's private jet. It was dark when we took off, and Ally and I went crazy trying to get him to tell us where we were going. An hour and a half later, the smell of hibiscus and bougainvillea and the soft moist air embraced us as we stepped off the plane. Bermuda. One of our favorite places. Ally jumped into his arms and slobbered him with kisses like a Lab puppy.

In addition, he had booked us into the Horizons hotel, where we had honeymooned 20 years before. Later that night I was luxuriating in the king sized bed, listening to the tropical birds, the whir of the wood fan, and the distant sound of the surf. I was just beginning to nod off. Peter came back from reading Ally a story and sat down next to me.

"So, do you remember?" he asked.

Uh-oh, I thought. It had been so long since we'd made love, I hadn't really expected it. "Yeah, well, I remember how to do it," I said, hoping humor might be a bit of a lubricant.

He laughed. "Hey, I just meant did you remember this was the very same room."

I flashed on that carried-over-the-threshold moment. "My God, you're right. I can't believe it. I'm sorry. I just didn't notice."

There was a slight flush of hurt on his face.

I realized that maybe he meant this whole trip was as much for me as for Ally. Maybe it was for us.

I reached for him. And we did remember.

I hated the thought that it had been mostly me keeping him at arm's length all these years. I thought of calling him up and offering to cook a late dinner, and then maybe.. . . But I quickly killed the impulse. He would have snacked at the office. The Bermuda trip was a long time ago. We hadn't been together that way since.

Ally. I couldn't get her out of my head. And I didn't even want to. My thoughts and memories were all I had left. It was two years, two months, thirteen days, and eighteen hours since Ally died. July 14, 2000. Bastille Day.

It had already been a rough sophomore year for her. Ally's old friend network had fractured as each of her pals hooked up with some guy. Ally was the only one who wasn't interested in guys yet, and her friends' obsessions about looks and boys bugged her. She was still a tomboy who would rather play sports and go backpacking than sit around listening to music and moaning over how much a Brad, Bill, or Bobby really cared.

Ally didn't talk to me about this, but I did pick up snippets from being the invisible chauffer on the trips to the mall. Most of our communication was in the form of arguments about what constitutes a picked-up room and enough studying for tests. Peter tried to be the referee, but we both told him to butt out.

I wanted us to try family therapy, but he was adamantly opposed. "You think the whole free world ought to be in therapy. She's 15. That's all we need to keep in mind. Wait till she gets her license. She'll feel better then. I certainly did when I was her age."

"Yeah, the license really helped, Peter," I once slashed at him a few months after the accident. He recoiled as if I'd slapped him, and I was shocked that even my hot temper could led me to be that cruel. But initially he'd been right. That spring she made varsity sailing and got her license. She was much better. I even overheard her telling a friend that there was a particular boy on her radar screen.

By summer Ally and Hank were inseparable and she was radiant. Like she was that last night.

She was wearing painted-on blue jeans and the low-cut pink tank top with a butterfly appliqué on the front, her mess of blonde hair pulled into a ponytail.

"For godsake, Ally, those jeans will cut off your circulation."

"Mom, you're clueless about styles. Look at what you have on."

I looked down at my outfit of Peter cast-offs; a white T-shirt and baggy khaki shorts. "Okay, so you've got a point. Just don't be such a smarty pants. And don't forget to be in by midnight."

"Whatever," she said, and banged the screen door behind her.

At 12:32 the phone rang.

"Mrs. Harney, there's been an accident and we need you to come down to Mt. Auburn hospital immediately."

"Is she okay?"

"I don't know, Ma'am," said the man. "Just come to the hospital."

Peter drove like a maniac while I cried hysterically, begging God, "Anything, anything, just let her be alive."

We barged through the revolving doors into the bright fluorescent white room.

I could tell from the huddle of doctors and nurses that turned to look at us.

When Peter came back down the hall from identifying her, he was staggering like a drunk. I ran to him. He couldn't look at me.

"Let me see her," I said, despite their warnings about how bad it was. I rushed toward the closed door behind him.

"No, Beth, don't. It's not the way to remember her."

I beat on his chest, screaming over and over "That's my daughter in there. I have to see my daughter." He held me tight till I gave up. I didn't want to leave her there at the hospital. He took me home.

I thought of her empty room upstairs. I didn't remember the rest. Later Peter told me that I went into the kitchen and started cooking fried eggs over easy and bacon with English muffins, Ally's favorite. I announced to him that an old-fashioned family breakfast was a fine idea.

There are no words. People who haven't been through it just don't get it. Like picking out the coffin, choosing hymns and prayers. I wanted Peter to do everything, but then I couldn't let him. The days were a blur of food, friends, tears, and murmurs. Everyone was trying so hard. Nothing helped.

"Beth, they're doing their best," Peter reminded me.

"I want them all to go away. I want my daughter back!"

He held me tight. I did better after that. But my heart turned to ice.

The phone rang again.

"What," I barked into it. I didn't care who was on the other end.

"Whoa there," said Peter. "Just calling to say that the meeting is over early and I'll be home in an hour. Maybe we could have dinner?"

"So now you tell me. Do you think I just stand around all day in my kitchen in a frilly apron waiting for dinner orders?"

"Lighten up, will you, Beth? You are such a pain in the ass."

I bit my tongue. He was so right.

"You win, your honor. Steak and béarnaise sauce with fries and asparagus, coming right up. The Judge Harney Special," I said sweetly, and surprisingly, even felt it a little. It had been a long time since I had cooked Peter's favorite meal.

I put down the phone and told myself to stop thinking about those last moments. . . . I had to hold onto the good memories. That's what Ally would want. I reached inside my desk drawer and pulled out my favorite picture. It was the one of Ally in the Optimist dinghy the day of her first solo sail. She was only seven.

Ally was so competent at everything about sailing. She had been quick to learn how to tie and splice, trim the sails, and take the helm. When she was only nine, she insisted on learning how to change the oil and fuel filters on the diesel of *Salient*, our old Bermuda 40 yawl. She even had Peter show her how to bleed the fuel lines. And she loved navigation. It was so easy for her to pick up dead reckoning as well as learn how to use the fancy instruments like Loran-C radionavigation and the new radar.

Peter had loved sailing since childhood despite its being such a snooty WASP sport. He had been captain of the sailing team at Milton. It was great for him that Ally took to it like the proverbial duck to water. I remembered another great picture we used to have. Ally standing on the seat holding the big wheel, frowning with concentration, and Peter right behind her; both of them scanning the compass, sail trim, and instruments. What a pair.

At the funeral, Peter got all the way through reading "To an Athlete Dying Young" without choking up, but his voice broke and his face contorted when he said, "Ally, my child, you will always be the light of our lives, the sparkle of gold on the rolling sea, now and forever. Fair winds, sailor."

My eyes were stinging. I was frozen to my office chair. I had to cook this special meal. But I couldn't put the picture down. Ally's smile glowed as the sail was catching the wind. She was in a white T-shirt and khaki shorts, enveloped by the orange life preserver. One hand on the tiller and the other waving at us. Her face was already turning away and looking up toward the sail when Peter had snapped the shot. The smile wasn't for us. It was clearly a burst of delight as the little boat came to life.

The Optimist picture was Peter's favorite, too. But he couldn't stand to see it. The old Monadnock picture of me nursing Ally as a baby was the only one he could tolerate around the house now. He had taken every other one down.

Peter wouldn't talk about her, and he refused therapy. I didn't push. I knew deep down he blamed himself. He'd minimized her experimenting with drugs and alcohol. "Don't be such a worrywart. All kids do this. I've talked with her about it. If she has too much she'll just sleep it off. She's promised she won't drive. What the hell, when I was her age, I remember driving home at 4:00 in the morning, tripping on acid. And we didn't even have seatbelts back then."

They found out later that Ally's blood alcohol level was off the charts.

I was so tired of gnawing on these memories, tired of thinking about Ally. And, honestly, sick and tired of Ally herself. The selfish brat. What was she thinking, getting into the car drunk?

"Being mad and even mad at the person who died is a natural part of healing," my therapist reminded me.

"I've said the same crap to my own clients, " I said back at her. "My daughter is dead and it's disgusting for me to be mad at her. It's sick."

The grieving went on and on. Every new season, holiday, any event was a reminder. Mornings were still the worst because I woke up having to remember. Sometimes she was so real in my dreams I'd thank God: She's okay and I've finally woken up from this crazy nightmare and everything was normal again. Then the alarm would go off. And I'd really wake up.

Peter said he didn't dream about her. That was for the best. He never wanted to talk about her, either. The one time he talked about it he said it felt like the old way of bleeding the boat's fuel lines. "After you change the fuel filter, you have to clear each section of line of the air bubbles because the engine will die out if there's any air in the line. In the old days, you'd suck the fuel through part of the line and then seal it off."

"But what did you do with the fuel in your mouth?"

"Well, that's the point. You just spat it into a bucket and were damned careful not to swallow any."

"Peter, pardon my obtuseness, but what's this procedure got to do with grief?"

"It's what I'm doing, Beth. Clearing each section of line bit by bit. Taking tiny sucks on the hose and trying not to swallow the fuel. Just trying to spit it all out."

I didn't really get it at the time, but sitting there and staring at Ally's smiling little face, I finally understood. Peter was right. I'd been poisoning myself by being so in touch with my damn feelings. I needed to blot things out. Compartmentalize like men do. I could only handle tiny sips of the memories and questions. This was too noxious. I was drowning in Ally.

"Just spit it out, Beth. Damn it. Just spit it out!" I said out loud in my empty office.

Suddenly, having a cold glass of Chardonnay while I cooked seemed like an inspirational idea.

Getting drunk was a bad idea. An hour and a half later, I was lying on the sofa with my third glass of wine, watching "Friends," Ally's favorite show. I might as well have been watching the clothes tumbling in the dryer. I had gotten dinner together, but Peter called very apologetically and said he'd be another half-hour. A little too cheerfully, I reassured him that dinner could wait and poured myself another glass. Somehow the sailing picture of Ally had ended up lying face down on my breast.

"Beth! Are you okay?" asked Peter. I must have dozed off. I sat up quickly, spilled some of my wine, and the picture frame fell to the floor.

"I'm okay. I'm sorry." I put the wine glass down on the coffee table. "I, uh, just had a little too much to drink, waiting for you, that's all."

But he wasn't listening. He was looking at Ally waving from the Optimist.

His face turned ashen.

"I thought we got rid of this." He bent over and picked it up.

"You can't erase her, Peter!"

"I just can't stand it."

"I'm sorry, I won't keep pretending she didn't exist. That's crazy."

"Thanks, Dr. Harney, is that what you tell all your patients?"

"You're not my client. You're my husband and you're her father."

"And you're fucking drunk, just like she was."

Peter raised the picture over his head and then smashed the frame over his knee, spewing shards of wood and glass all over the rug. He slid to the floor, his face twisted into a grimace. He groaned like a wounded animal.

My heart broke open. I knelt beside him and put my arms around him. He sobbed uncontrollably.

For a moment he let me just hold him. Then he whispered, "You know, it's my fault. I should have been tougher with her. She would have listened to . . . " and then he started crying again. I cradled his head in my arms, stroked his hair, and rocked him. I was crying, too.

On the rug, I glimpsed the crumpled picture of Ally in the broken frame. She was smiling up at us.

QUESTIONS FOR DISCUSSION

1. Is the way Peter and Beth deal with their daughter's death typical or unusual?

2. Many couples end up divorcing after the death of a child. Why would this be true? Is it inevitable?

3. Peter and Beth centered their lives on being parents and didn't address some of their unresolved marital issues. Whose fault was that? How did this affect their way of grieving?

4. All of us have experienced some difficult losses. How have you dealt with yours? What has helped and what hasn't? What are the key elements of dealing with loss and grief?

5. Twelve years after reconciling, Peter and Beth suddenly lose their only child. How do you feel about what's happened to them? How do you deal with the unpredictability and uncertainty in your life?

6. How might a couple of a different race, cultural group, or social class go through their grieving process? What might be difficult for a couple with significant differences in their cultural background?

THE MORNING
OF FEBRUARY FIFTH

Ann ran down the long corridors of an old Victorian mansion. Portraits of snarling men stared down at her as she raced by, holding her skirts up. Every time she reached a room she would throw open the heavy mahogany door and search wildly for any sign of Eliza. The rooms were always empty, yet somewhere down one of the corridors a terrible thing was being done to Eliza. She ran down the endless corridors from room to room, knowing she'd be too late.

She woke up. It was still black out, but she caught sight of the thin slice of the setting moon out of the corner of her window. Her moon. John was snoring away next to her. The clock read 5:05.

"Today is the first day of the rest of your life." She chuckled silently. A surge of electrical energy crackled through her. It was amazing that she slept at all. Now she was wide awake, ready and sure. She turned over on her side and noticed that telltale full feeling in her belly. Today of all days. But then it seemed bizarrely appropriate, her womb weeping blood.

Spare me the melodrama, "womb weeping" and what not, she thought. "Hey, that's no way, to say good-bye." Song lines had been flashing though her head ever since she had stopped her medication.

Better than hearing made-up voices. Everything had been easier when she was just a regular alcoholic. The second hospitalization, where they pumped her full of diagnoses, medications, and shock treatment was the one that almost killed her. That was when she had the flashbacks about what her father had done to her. Boy, that stuff made "The Game" with Dave pretty tame. She shuddered and closed her eyes and prayed for the strength to see her through.

But what about Max? He'd be trapped in the house all day. He'd wait as long as he could, whimpering by her bedside, but eventually he'd have to make a mess somewhere.

Ann slipped silently out of the bed. She had a pee, put in her tampon, and didn't flush. A glimpse in the mirror betrayed her fat rolls and her pendulous breasts that sagged toward her broad expanse of belly. Well past Rubenesque. She grimaced and looked around at the paraphernalia of self-care, body grooming, and beauty products on the toilet tank, around the sink, and in the cabinet above. She snuck back into the bedroom and hurriedly grabbed for sweatpants and a turtleneck. It was too dark to tell if they matched. As she tugged the pants up over her hips, she thought of John's not-so-subtle Christmas gift of the health club membership, and the "screw you" 20 pounds she had put on since then. To think that once upon a time she'd kept her perfect figure even if it did mean occasionally sticking her finger down her throat after any big meal, afraid of putting on an ounce. Now I'm on the ultimate diet plan, she thought, and smiled. You do have to be a little whacked to be doing this.

"Max," she whispered in his ear, and he was up instantly. "Shssh, sweetie," she said as she petted his head.

"What's up?" mumbled John.

"Nothing, I just couldn't sleep. I'm taking Max for a little pre-dawn walk. I'll wake you up when I get back."

"Is the alarm set?"

"John, go back to sleep. It's okay. I don't want you to miss your flight anymore than you do."

He rolled over, and Ann couldn't tell if he had even noticed the edge in her voice. She and Max padded downstairs. He was excited.

It had been a long time since there had been any early morning walks. She ground some high-octane espresso even though she knew after-dinner coffee for breakfast would annoy John. Oh well. Then she went over to the cupboard and got out some Alpo for Max. He'd get a treat of a full can today. She reached into the fridge and chose the heavy cream over the one percent. My, my, aren't we being a bad girl, and she felt the power surge in her brain. She wasn't right in the head. She didn't want to be.

Then she noticed the pictures on the door of the refrigerator: Chris at graduation, then Eliza standing between her and John, dressed up for some occasion. She looked even fatter in pictures than she did in the mirror. There was John, Chris, and Eliza on their skis on the top of Killington. They were all beaming. They'll be okay, she reassured herself.

She had thought a lot about them in the previous weeks. Those two children had been her rationale for slogging along for years. "You've got to remember how devastated the kids would be," Dr. Evans always used to say. "It's not just about you, Ann." And of course he orchestrated that intervention with John and then got poor Eliza and Chris to beg her to stop drinking. That bastard. She never should have confessed everything to him in the first place. His guilt-trip technique had worked for years, but they had never really talked about what happens when the kids grow up. What would he use to tie her down now? He'd probably do another intervention and pop her into another hospital.

Max raced though his food and was jumping up and down at the front door. She reached for his leash on one of the hooks that held all their coats in the back hall. Chris's and Eliza's ski parkas were still there, just as if they were still in high school.

"Come on, Max," she whispered, and stepped into the cold darkness.

The morning twilight, she called it, and she looked up at the sky to see if it was still dark enough to catch a glimpse of the North Star. There it was. She was cold but it didn't bother her. She remembered how much she treasured these walks: stolen moments away from family and the chaotic rush through making lunches and launching children. Max tugged at his leash and yanked her forward. Only a thin parallel line of car tracks marred the white expanse. The snow squeaked under her feet. Last tracks, she thought, and again was taken with her sense of cold clarity and conviction.

Dawn's light slowly brought the shapes around her into focus, the big pines in front of the Clarks' house, the road stretching ahead of her, the looming hulk of Fisk Hill ahead. She wouldn't walk far. Max was sniffing and doing his business all over the place, emphatically claiming the neighborhood as his territory. She should have been a dog.

When Ann and Max returned, John was dressed and at the kitchen table. He was pouring more milk into his coffee.

"Christ, Ann, this stuff will put you on the ceiling. Why didn't you make the half and half?"

"I just felt in need of an extra jolt today. Sorry." She bent over the dishwasher to hide her smile. "What time will you be home tonight?"

"Late." He got up and headed for the coat rack. "Don't hold supper for me."

She walked around to the back hall just as he opened the door. "Well, have a good day."

He didn't catch her forced smile. "You, too," he called back over his shoulder, and closed the door behind him.

The minute he left, she went back upstairs and yanked off her clothes and threw them on the floor. She put her flannel nightgown back on and wrapped herself in her warm, fuzzy pink bathrobe. She reached into her nightstand and pulled out the brown paper bag. It hadn't taken her any time at all to accumulate enough. She had both her psychiatrist and her internist giving her Ambien for sleep, Xanax for her anxiety, Depakote for her mood disorder, and Seroquel for her thought disorder. And she had simply stopped taking them.

The little handful of daily meds had kept her pinned like a butterfly. She'd known what would happen if she stopped taking them. She'd be completely out of her mind. And she was. She felt like herself again. It had been a long time.

It was tough keeping it together now that she'd "gone over the wall," as they say. She spilled out onto the bedspread her stash of multihued pills: all her pretty little prison guards, now the means of her own "Great Escape." She counted out a mix of 60 pills. She was a little worried about throwing them up, but she'd take them slowly, but not so slowly that she passed out too soon. She had decided on eight at once with milk.

But first the notes. What could she possibly say? Words trivialize everything. But not to write, particularly to Chris and Eliza, would be even more of a slap in the face to her children. And if she wrote them then obviously she'd have to write to John.

She got up and put on Eliza's bunny slippers and padded back downstairs to the kitchen. She went over to her mother's Federal period writing desk. It was an expensive antique of glossy mahogany wood with strips of gold inlay. Her mother gave it to her one Christmas along with a box of monogrammed stationery: "You can use it for your overdue thank you notes, Dearie," said her mother with her arch chuckle.

She had never sat at it before. It had always simply been for decoration, providing a hint of elegance to an otherwise drab and conventional suburban kitchen. It belonged in her mother's new house, where everything matched perfectly. She bought it after Ann's father died and her mother cleaned up her act. Her mother stopped drinking all on her own, and now she and her brother, Dave, simply pretended like nothing bad had ever happened. They talked about Dad as if he had a "little too much stress" and that's why he had an "anger management problem"—her mother's words. It made her want to punch her lights out. Except obviously Mother didn't have any lights on, thought Ann, and shook her head.

Dave's denial hurt much worse. Once she asked him if he remembered them cuddling up with each other when the parents were fighting and he looked at her like she was crazy. Well, she might be crazy, but not about that.

Ann rummaged through the desk and found the unopened box. The stationery was a thick, cream-colored linen paper with a dashing letterhead. She took out a sheet and placed it on the green blotter. It looked blank and beautiful. She pulled the pen from the penholder and paused to look out into the backyard at the snow-covered branches of the magnolia and the shroud of snow hiding the disarray of her lawn and gardens that she hadn't really tended to at all in the last couple of years. It started to snow again.

She didn't know whom to start with. John seemed the easiest. She sighed and then bent over the page.

From the desk of Ann Symington

February 5, 2003

Dear John,

Well, here goes, even though I know you'll never understand and there really isn't any point. It just seems like the right thing to do, to write to you and say whatever I can.

This isn't meant to hurt you and (don't take this personally) it isn't even about you. In the end, it's just an is.

But I see you coming home tonight and it seems best that you should read this before coming up and discovering the remains.

Ann paused and decided she would leave letters, each in their own separate envelope, right out on the kitchen table so he couldn't miss seeing them.

I know that it doesn't really soften the blow and I don't mean to be mean.

Ann looked up from the page. Damn, this was going to be hard. She felt the power surge draining out of her and forced herself back to the page.

John wouldn't understand any of this.

So, anyway, here I am, John, a wife, the children, the soccer mom, the shelter volunteer, and now, supposedly to fill the dreaded empty nest, I'm supposed to be a social worker, a surrogate mom to the inner children of "clients." Spare me. Spare them, too.

Listen, do me one favor. Some well-meaning grief counselor is bound to want you and the children to share your letters. Well, let the condemned have one last request. I'm going to write what I want to write in this letter. What I write to the children will be the best I can do for them. This is for me, John. Let it be between us. We never protected the children enough before. I'll never forgive you for telling the kids about everything the last time when you and Evans threw me into Westwood Lodge, on the borderlines from hell unit. It was bad enough with the intervention and having to go to AA. Hi, I'm Ann. I'm an alcoholic and all that. But that second time, just because I had said a few things about life not being worth living and cutting my wrist a little. For Chrissake it wasn't necessary to panic and throw me in the damn loony bin. I was still stone sober! And don't get me started on the shock therapy.

I didn't expect this to sound so pissed. They said in one of my courses that suicide is an act of rage as well as despair and all the mental illness crap. Well, duh! But seriously, I want to tell you the truth, but there's lots that the children don't need to know the details about. Like your recent male menopause philandering that you're stupid enough to think I don't know about. Frankly, my dear, it was actually a load off my mind that you were getting "it" elsewhere. Now I don't have to take your constant complaints about my weight even slightly seriously. But, honestly, I have been offended by the notion of you and Sheila in our bed. And don't ask how I figured that out.

Ann pushed back from the desk. She didn't like her nasty vindictive tone. It just doesn't really belong in this letter, she thought. Bimbos in motels had been bad enough, but having to sit through Sheila's tearful confession about her and John was a little more than she could take. But John, "you probably think this song is about you." Good old Carly Simon. Ann smiled and got up to get some more coffee.

So I'm back. I wanted to calm myself down. Anyway, one other thing. The imagined grief counselor (I think her name will be Bloom, Mrs. Bloom, not a Dr. Bloom, just a Mrs.). (Please don't drag everyone in to see Evans. I suspect he will take this very hard.) Anyway, Mrs. Bloom will undoubtedly try to help all of you understand that this is not your fault and is the result of my many mental illnesses, like my depression or my manic–depression, or my alcoholism, or my so-called PTSD.

Well, the children can believe whatever they need to in order to relieve their guilt. It really isn't their fault. But between you and me, the truth is that I'm no more mentally ill than my big fat matronly butt.

Actually, I haven't felt this good in years. You know when I decided. It was during the dessert at Christmas dinner, as all of you gorged on my sugar cookies, almond tortes, and the peppermint ice cream with my homemade chocolate sauce. I looked at all of you and knew (as I nibbled on my one little cookie because after all I am way too fat and lately I've heard obesity can be life threatening, ha ha) "this could be the last time, this could be the last time, maybe the last time, I don't know, oh no."

Ann stopped dead. I can't exactly claim that I'm totally sane and than lapse into stupid humor and silly song riffs. She looked at the page. The thought of starting over was impossible and crossing stuff out seemed ridiculously messy. She was just going to have to keep a lid on it. And she wasn't about to tell him that she had a few sips of Scotch that night, which was her first taste in 14 years. Or that she had been sneaking drinks ever since then. None of it was any of his damn business.

I'm exhausted. I'm going to rest a bit and then try to write Eliza. She's going to be the hardest hit anyway. I'm not that worried about Chris. He may be younger but he's really a chip off the old block. He'll get through it okay. I'm just hoping that Robert will help Eliza through. He's a good kid and you can tell how much he loves her. All through Christmas, I watched him watch her. He adores her.

Do you remember the first Christmas with my family and the love poem you read to me at the table? It was the happiest moment in my life. Well, one of them, anyway. I think I'd have to put holding Eliza in my arms for the first time first. Oh, I don't know.

Ann reached up and ran her fingers through her hair. It was greasy and thick with too much buildup of hairspray. But a shower seemed quite superfluous. She got up to stretch. Max looked up hopefully from his bed in the kitchen.

She sat back down at the desk and pulled the photo album from her bottom drawer. There they were in all the ages and stages; John and her walking down the aisle, impossibly young, looking like children in dress-up clothes, her holding Eliza, birthday parties, graduations, trips, and on and on.

The wetness on her cheeks surprised her. A cigarette suddenly seemed like a brilliant idea. Never mind she hadn't smoked in five years. She had saved a pack in the back of her closet in case of emergencies.

She went to retrieve an ashtray from the liquor cabinet. She paused as she looked at the array of gleaming bottles. A drop or two of Glenlivet in her coffee seemed like a fine idea, too. She just had to make sure she didn't have too much. She couldn't lose her focus, and sometimes booze made her a little maudlin. That wouldn't do. Besides, John would check the bottle later and it was the last thing she wanted him to be able to blame it on.

The first drags seared her lungs and, combined with the first sip, she felt light-headed. What the hell, she shrugged, and pulled out a fresh piece of paper.

From the desk of Ann Symington

Dear Eliza,

I hear your great grandfather's clock ticking. Outside our kitchen window, the snowflakes are the size of butterflies and they are lightly landing on the limbs of the magnolia. Do you remember us planting that tree together—one of those endless Girl Scout projects? You were so disappointed that you had to wait a whole year for the flowers to come, and then those impossibly large pink blossoms that seemed as big artichokes and how excited you were and then how quickly they fell.

I just started looking at our albums. You were always the one for making me sit down and take the time to put the pictures together. I was always "too busy," but you used to B&B (remember "beg and badger"?) me till you wore me out: "But, Mommy, they're for making forever happen."

Ann grimaced. Eliza would be reading this afterwards. It was all too treacly sweet. What if she got inspired to read some of it at the service? Max was barking at the door. Of course, Mr. Campbell with the dry cleaning. She heard him come in the back hall and didn't move a muscle when he called out, "Anything for me today, Missus?" Then she heard the door slam. She'd have to remember to lock the door. Now back to work.

Eliza, let me cut to the chase. There's nothing sweet or sentimental about what I'm about to do. I'm going to murder your mother in cold blood. It's a premeditated act that would probably get me the death penalty if I were around for it (sorry, poor attempt at humor).

Eliza, here's my problem. I can't explain it so that it will make sense. I can't expect you to understand. I've been hanging on for dear life since I was little, and truth is I'm just too sick and tired of being sick and tired and all the pretend. I am glad that you and Chris helped me stop drinking when you were only eight, and I remember how sweet your letter was that you read at the intervention and I can't tell you how many times I read it over. It was so brave of you to stand up to me when I was such a mess. And I remember standing by your bed my first night back from the hospital and promising that I would be there for you no matter what until "you were grown and safely on your way" (as the song from some musical says). It worked. The last 14 years haven't been so bad. But even though I promised myself to not pick up a drink, I really never got better. I just "acted as if," like they say in AA. It really wasn't until that second time in the hospital that I knew this day might come and that—well, you were about ten then—I would wait till you were more grown up. Then I would know when it was time to go, then I could finally choose for me. And so here I am, sweetie, and it is a choice and in my heart I know it's the right choice.

Of course, you have a right to be angry. This is unbelievably selfish. And if you and Robert ever have children, they will only have one grandmother, but Mrs. McIntyre does seems nice. Anyway, we're all going to die and my time simply has come sooner than expected. It could have been a brain tumor. I do have a diseased mind, after all (sorry, not funny).

The most important thing, and I hope Robert is there with you as you read this and if not, go get him now or wait for him.

Eliza, my first born, love of my life, light of my light. It is not your fault.

I am so sorry. There are really no excuses. I just have to go. Please know how much I love you. Please trust me on that.

> *I love you,*
> *Mom*

P.S. If you really have to know about my demons, then contact Dr. Jack Evans, my old shrink. You met him back when you were little. He will fill in the blanks for you. He knows details about my childhood that nobody else knows. And he knows how hard I tried. I haven't seen him for years, but he did understand me.

P.P.S. Bye, sweetie.

Ann closed her eyes. She reached for another tissue and another cigarette. They were making her dizzy and a little nauseous, like morning sickness. Was this mourning sickness? "Oh, Ann," she winced. She stubbed out the cigarette. She realized the rank smell of smoke would be one of John's first clues. It might be a small kindness.

Max was scratching at the door. The cleaner had obviously let him out. She opened the door and said, "Hi, there, Max, looks like we're both having a busy day."

She wanted a nap. But now to Chris.

From the desk of Ann Symington

February 5, 2003

Dear Chris,

I've already written Eliza, but this isn't getting any easier.

I think of you as the big maple in our backyard spreading out to the sky in all directions. You tower over the rest of us. Your trunk is thick and solid, unyielding, unbendable, and your roots are dug so deep into Mother Earth. I pray I'm right about you. You're the baby, but I believe you'll be okay. You've always been the steady one, the watcher. When you were about five and your dad and I had all those fights, before they packed me off to the treatment center, Eliza would be crying and getting in between us and there you'd be on the back stairs, just watching. Just like you were watching "The Simpsons." Remember how I used to call you the Littlest Baby Buddha? You always had this calm, inscrutable face with just the slightest hint of a smile.

I know this will wound you too. But somehow I hope you'll know that none of this is your fault. Just keep on keeping on. Do the guy thing. I often wish that I had been a boy. Maybe I could have kept the lid on Pandora's box with a little bit of good old-fashioned masculine compartmentalization. Which isn't to say that I think you're cold, unfeeling, or disconnected. I know you have a kind and tender heart. You just seem so contained. I know you'll know that what I want for you is to keep going on with your life, and that includes Berlin next semester. Such a great opportunity to really perfect your German and learn so much more about those dour philosophers you love so much. I just Kant make any sense of them, but the Hegel with it. (Sorry, Mom's punning again.)

Undoubtedly you'll become the department protégé. Or, who knows, maybe you'll Nietzsche all that and become a venture capitalist or, God forbid, a therapist. Sorry, Chris, I know there's no jest in this gesture. I can't help it. You always got my cockeyed sense of humor. I just don't want you to let this mess slow you down. Silly me. I know that I'm wanting to soften the blow.

Chris, I know that there's no easing of the pain through my words. I used to think I didn't matter and everyone would be better off without me. But thanks to the miracle of therapy, I know that I matter and that my doing this will scar you.

Forgive me for not giving you and Eliza the chance to talk me out of this. I'm not that strong, and then where would I be? In another hospital, biding my time so that the next time would be the last time. And what's the good in that, Chris?

Please, my darling boy, just know that there really was nothing you could do and it's not your fault. It was your turn to leave the nest, not mine, but the Mommy bird has to go. Please let me go.

I'm holding the picture of you in your Doctor Denton's baby pajamas and me in my evening dress; we are bending toward each other for a good-night kiss. You must have been about four. Before the crazy times. I loved you so much. I always have. I always will.

Mom

Ann heard the rattle outside and looked at the big gray squirrel hanging upside down between the bars to get at the bird feed. They really should call it a squirrel feeder, Ann thought, and shook her head. Nature's way. Squirrel wins.

She needed a breath of fresh air and pushed open the back door through the snow. There was at least six inches now. She lit another cigarette, took another sip of her Scotch-laced coffee, and stood for a moment with her slippers and ankles buried in the snow and thought, just finish the letter to John.

From the desk of Ann Symington

John, I've just written the kids. They don't deserve this and it rips me to pieces. You know we put them (no, correction) I put them through so much. You did try. You did hang in there with me when I was a complete nut case. You held the family together. I get that. But it's been 14 years. And I've done the best I could, too.

So you've started doing your thing, and who can blame you. I know I'm no prize. And now the empty nest will be all yours. Anyway, the real point is the kids are going to need you even more than before, and just because they're older and act okay doesn't really mean they will be. Get them help, John. Promise me that.

I am truly sorry. You didn't really deserve any of this either.

A

P.S. Please don't share this letter with the kids. I really don't want them to know about Sheila. They like her.

"Done!" she said out loud, and pushed her bulky body away from the chair. Max barked. She looked at the sheets of pages neatly stacked one on top of another. Just drivel, she thought. She folded her arms and hugged herself. She felt chilled to the bone. Gone was the snap, crackle, and pop. So were the tears. She was just tired, and stood blankly looking out the window at the snow coming down heavily.

Suddenly she felt ravenous for a cheese omelet. She started bustling about the kitchen. Her energy surged back. She knew she better not take any more sips, even to wash down the other stuff. This was definitely "controlled drinking" as they call it, and she smiled. She thought of what she needed to get at the store later, before she caught herself. She gave Max a bite of egg. She realized there really had to be another letter.

After a very satisfying breakfast and a trip to the john, she sat back down, reached for another piece of stationery from the box, and picked up her pen. She felt ready to write again.

From the desk of Ann Symington

February 5, 2003

Dr. Evans,

This is an apology note, a thank you note, and a forgiveness note, plus, you know, that other kind of note. I remember your office, the bright splash of light on your red Oriental rug, your desk behind you piled with junk, the big easy chair that made me feel so little.

So. Where to start? Your cherry rocking chair that you pulled over to me so that you could sit close to me. I remember you leaning toward me, and your kind eyes. They were so gentle and held me so tenderly. You were more of a mother to me than anyone else has ever been.

Anyway, enough of the warm fuzzies. It's just that if it weren't for you, I wouldn't have been able to see my kids grow up. Yes, I'm thanking you for the damn intervention that I was mad about, and even the trip to the nut house. It's true. I wouldn't be alive today without that. You made me know how important I was. You helped my kids get through to me, and it worked. I'm glad I did. And you'll be pleased to know that I was a pretty good mom, too. I mean not entirely, especially after the ECT zapped the hell out of me. But I baked the brownies, made Halloween costumes, checked the homework, and patrolled the sidelines of every single one of their games. You do understand I couldn't have done all that if I had kept coming in to see you. I had to put the lid on it. I mean, I hope you didn't take that personally. I just couldn't talk anymore about what happened to me when I was little.

Anyway, I'm sure someone will call you and you'll know before you get this. Just please don't think that you did something wrong back then. I did the best I could. Then and now. I wouldn't be surprised if John or Eliza calls you. Tell them whatever might be helpful.

And please understand that you truly saved my life (for which I have been occasionally ungrateful) but I do thank you for it.

Anyway, Doc, just don't beat yourself up, okay?

Be well,

Ann

Ann put the cap back on the fountain pen, then paused, opened it again and carefully addressed each envelope: *John, Eliza, Chris,* then *Dr. Evans.* She carefully folded each letter and stuffed it in. She licked each envelope. Outside, the snow had turned to a drizzle. She pushed away from the desk and put the stack of envelopes on the kitchen counter. She headed upstairs. Max followed, wagging his tail.

QUESTIONS FOR DISCUSSION

1. Given what you know about Ann and her history, why do you think she decided to commit suicide at this time in her life? Was it inevitable?
2. Ann is aware that by going off her medication and beginning to drink again, she was putting herself at risk for becoming manic or psychotic. Was her suicide an act of free will or a manifestation of insanity, or both?
3. Retrospectively, it appears that Evans shifted from being her individual therapist to doing an alcohol intervention and collaborating with her husband in hospitalizing her when she appeared suicidal. Was this a mistake?

4. If the therapy with Evans had been somehow different, might it have prevented Ann's suicide? How? Why?
5. In her letters to her children, Ann is trying to help them through their pain about her suicide. Would these letters help? What would be the range of feelings you might have if you were Ann's child, husband, or therapist?
6. Have you ever lost a client, friend, or family member to suicide? What was your experience and what helped you get through it?

THE AMERICAN
CAB COMPANY

"Never again will we be surprised by the forces of evil. If Saddam won't give up his weapons of mass destruction then we have to go into Iraq to protect our precious American way of life." Jack can hear Bush pounding the podium somewhere in Iowa, Heartland country.

He glances at the thickening traffic, all the commuters in huge gas-guzzling sport utility vehicles named after tribes like Cherokee and Comanche. These SUVs aren't fording rivers or climbing mountains. They're slowing to a rush hour crawl on the Schuylkill Expressway.

"Yep, we definitely need that oil," Jack says inadvertently out loud.

"You got that right, man," says the cabbie. "We've got to kick some serious Arab butt. Force is the only thing those people respect."

"Sure," says Jack. He can't resist asking "And so, what do you think of his tax cuts?"

The fat, bald cabbie turns around and gives Jack the eye, as if he's no longer sure whether he's talking to a friend or foe. "Ya know, the whole thing is you got to get people spending money. The stupid government just takes it and wastes it. Ever since 9/11, nobody is spending money, not the big guys on Wall Street or the little guys at the mall. Bush just wants to get the whole thing going again, kind of like jump-starting a car battery."

Jack smiles. He was planning on using the jump-start metaphor in his workshop on intimacy today. So much for ownership of ideas. He glances at his watch. Damn. It's almost 8 A.M. He should be thinking about the workshop rather than debating with the cabbie. Jack looks at the photo ID card and discovers he's been debating with Lou Abrizzi and he's riding in the American Cab Company, no less. Jack shakes his head.

"Yep," says Lou, as he slows to take an exit, "It's people spending money that makes this good old U.S. of A. work."

Lou sounds a lot like Skipper, and he hears his dad's voice from a recent late night phone call. "Listen, Jackie boy, you liberals don't know shit about when it's time to step up to the plate. You get all the benefits of our armed forces doing what they have to do but you don't want to pay the price."

Jack sighed. Dad's been in the sauce again.

"Besides, all you people do is talk. If you feel so strongly about this, Jacko, why aren't you doing something like writing your congressman or doing one of those stupid protest marches you used to do when you were a kid?"

Jack knew better than to argue with his dad when he was in his cups, and part of him even agreed with the old man. He does just do the "talk the talk" bit. Voting had been his only demonstration of social activism for years. He remembers the lines:

> And you will have on a nice suit
> With matching tie and wife
> Color-coordinated children
> And a nice, good life.

They were written by his angry, self-righteous 21-year-old self about how he would turn out by the time he was 40 (and that seemed terminally old back then).

Jack looks around at the other commuters inching their way into the city and thinks maybe he has been "co-opted by the system," as they used to say.

Back during the peak of his involvement in radical politics he had had the startling realization that fighting "the system" had become for him a self-centered way to prove himself. Taking on the U.S. government was simply an extension of battling with his dad. Then at 22, he walked away from the Cause and went to graduate school to become a therapist. He decided that he needed the direct emotional connection to the people he was trying to help. That would be the way he would make a difference.

Recently, Jack has been feeling like a fraud even in his clinical work. Sometimes he feels like he's just a "rent-a-friend." People come to him for an emotional fix just like they have makeovers done at the spa. Consumers spending money chasing happiness makes the country great. Just ask his new pal, Lou Abrizzi.

Outside the office, he didn't have much left over for his community, his friends, or even his wife and kids. Someday he would like to say to his father, "Yes, it's true. I'm not on the barricades anymore, but I believe in what I do. I'm not living in a grandiose revolutionary abstraction, but here, now, just trying to be a good-enough husband, father, therapist, one person, one moment at a time."

Skipper would snort at this. Jack realizes he's never going to try having that sort of conversation with his dad again. They're both too old now. And he isn't really sure it is a good-enough life. Or that he's very good at it. Maybe the self-righteous, know-it-all poet was on the money. Jack wonders if it's time to check back in with his old therapist, Beth. He doesn't even know if she is still in practice. He misses seeing her.

Then he thinks of Ann's suicide note. Ann assumed he would have heard the news before reading it. But, no, he got it directly from her. Sadly enough, it wasn't a shock. When he saw her stationery, his first thought was it's "the note." What she said didn't surprise him either. He never really understood why getting sober and going to AA hadn't worked for her. He suspected there was probably much more trauma history, and maybe even sexual abuse at the hands of her raging father, than he had ever realized. Besides, the whole way he worked with her back then felt off. He didn't really have any business opening up her trauma history the way he did without helping her develop better coping skills. And he certainly should have recognized that doing the intervention with her husband and her kids would wreck their individual therapy, but he didn't know what else to do once he found out how much she was drinking.

Jack winces as the would'ves, could'ves, and should'ves sting him like angry hornets.

The cab jerks to a stop just as they get into downtown Philadelphia. They're still a ways from the conference center. Time to concentrate on his presentation.

*   *   *

Just five blocks ahead of Jack, Mary O'Donnell is also stuck in the traffic. "I'm too old for this," she sighs as she tries to keep one eye on the red light while tracing a thin black line across her eyelid. She's not exactly sure what she's too old for: being late and putting on makeup in traffic, or going to another workshop in order to keep up her CEU's, and one on sex, intimacy, and grief to boot.

"But Karen," she'd said, "I don't even treat couples. You know most of my clients are abuse survivors.

"Well, maybe that's what he means by the grief part. I just hear the guy is good. Supposedly, he makes a daylong go by in the blink of an eye. Besides, the brochure says that it isn't just about technique. He's also going to talk about how therapists deal with their own issues around this stuff." Karen was always keen on therapists being supportive of each other and talking openly about their own struggles.

"God, Karen, it sounds like a touchy-feely, sharing enterprise. Spare me."

"Come on, kiddo, you know us therapists are just as screwed up as everyone else."

"Well, I'm not going to 'share' as they say, but if it will shut you up, I'll come," said Mary. She wasn't about to acknowledge that she was a little curious.

129

She adjusts the mirror so she can put on some lipstick.

It does bother her that Frank never reaches for her anymore, and anytime she brings it up he seems to shrink away from the whole subject. What do other women do? Which brings her back to the "too old" question. Here she is in the middle of hot flashes and HRT and worrying about whether her husband is interested. Not that she's necessarily interested herself, but it really bothers her that he isn't. She remembers back to when they both couldn't get enough and all the years after the kids came along when it was just him that couldn't get enough. Every time she turned around there he was, like a big Newfoundland puppy, a slobbering a mess of friendly affection and wheedling neediness, pawing all over her. "Huh, huh? How about it, tonight? What do you say, huh?" He was never going to be a writer for Hallmark cards.

"After the day I've had. You've got to be kidding," she would invariably respond.

And sure enough he would slink off and she'd feel bad and promise herself that they'd do it tomorrow and just wish it wasn't always such a big deal with him. And now he could care less. Of course, with Jason being home, they didn't have time for anything but worrying about him, anyway. Jason's such a mess with his piercings, shaved head, and bleary-eyed pothead bewilderment. If only Frank didn't coddle him so much. They've got to confront the drug stuff. Mary hates the way Jason wheedles money out of them with one pathetic excuse after another. Her baby. The druggie dropout.

Finally the light turns green.

*   *   *

Mary looks around at the packed room at the Holiday Inn. All ages and all stages. Dressed up–dressed down. Eager–bored. Mellow–tense. There isn't a spare chair and it's already hot. People are fanning themselves and shifting around in their seats uncomfortably. It's only 9:00. Mary uses her program for a fan. "Phew, it's going to be a long day," she says to Karen, who is already pulling off her navy

Shetland sweater, the one with the reindeer racing across her front and the snowflakes on the shoulders. It's the one she wears to workshops with her old tattered jeans, which always makes Mary wonder why she dresses up for these things. She glances down at her teal business suit and matching pumps.

"Listen, Mary, I know I dragged you here, but, really, you can't complain all day. You'll drive me crazy," says Karen, who's now patting her curly hair back into some semblance of order.

Mary says, "Okay, Sister, I'll be good." And she straightens her back, presses her knees together, and folds her hands in her lap as if she were a novitiate.

Karen laughs, and then they are hushed by Sandra Kellerman, who's introducing Evans.

After the applause dies down, Mary checks out Evans as he walks to the podium.

She notes his formal dark blue suit and red power tie. "At least he dresses well, she whispers to Karen and then settles back into the seat, trying to make herself comfortable.

"Listen, before I get started," starts Evans, "Can we get the heat turned down a little? After all, we are going to be talking about sex and it could get a little hot in here."

The audience titters and some applaud.

"You know, it's much easier to talk about our clients than ourselves, but I think it's impossible to work with couple issues around intimacy and sexuality without paying attention to our stuff. I'm not going to stand up here and just blather on about me all day. We are all going to learn from each other. Let me start with a personal question."

"So, how many of you have had, are having, or would like to have a sex life?"

The group bursts into laughter and everyone raises their hands.

Mary looks over at Karen and rolls her eyes.

"And how many of you are completely satisfied with your sexual and intimate life?"

Nobody raises their hands.

"Actually," he goes on, "the trick word in the question is 'completely.' All of us struggle with the problem of what's good enough: good-enough money, good-enough relationship, good-enough sex. In this culture, we're always thinking more will be better and that we deserve to be happy. Like it's one of the inalienable rights in the Declaration of Independence. However, before I go on a rant about our materialist culture, let's focus."

Evans pauses and walks around the front of the podium with his handheld mike. He softens his voice. "I do have one more question."

Uh-oh, thinks Mary.

"How many of you have experienced a profound loss or grief in your life? I don't mean just by death. I'm talking about all our losses and disappointments: marriages failing, kids struggling, our dashed dreams, getting older, friendships ending. I mean all the losses of life. How many of you carry a deep grief?"

All the hands in the audience go up. The room is very still.

"Yes," Evan says gently, "all of us, each of us in our own way, know what it means to have a broken heart. Today is not just about techniques for treating our clients' intimacy issues. It's also about the core grief we carry and how that plays out in our own intimate lives and in our clinical work."

"But let's not start there; it's way too heavy. First let me pair you up to deal with some specific questions about sexuality and intimacy. I always get some negative feedback from a few folks who really don't come to a workshop to talk to the people sitting next to them. Well, give it a try. Sometimes we have more to learn from and more to teach each other than we give ourselves credit for."

Mary turns to Karen.

"So, what did ya think?" asks Karen with a big smile. She's obviously already taken with the guy.

"Personally, he seems a little too smooth and a little too self-satisfied, says Mary, "And I hate these kind of instant connection type exercises. Anyway, what was our question?"

"We're supposed to talk about how our personal experience affects our work with couples."

"I don't know how you got me here. You go first."

Karen smiles and says, "Honestly, I like working with this stuff.

I'd rather talk about sex than whose turn it is to clean up the kitchen. I mean, it can be tough because the guys in my practice sometimes think it's automatically two against one, but usually I can get them to loosen up. They always like it when I turn to their wives and say, 'Honey, you know, sometimes, you have to just 'put out.' "

"Come on, Karen, you don't really say that, do you? Thank God you're not my therapist."

"No, seriously, I think if I hadn't been such a romantic about it all and so critical of Henry for just wanting to get laid, maybe we would have made it. Sometimes I think we expect too much of them. They're just guys, after all. Anyway, now it's your turn."

"Well, I don't know what to say. The place where this comes up in my practice is that once my clients have gotten in touch with having been sexually abused, most of them stop being able to be sexual at all and have a really strong PTSD response to their husband's sexuality. They just lock up."

"You don't want to talk about your own stuff, huh?" asks Karen with a raised eyebrow.

"No, I don't, and thanks for not taking the rather obvious hint, my dear friend. Anyway, I wonder if he's going to talk about any of the trauma stuff?"

"Ask him."

"Karen, lighten up, will you please?" whispers Mary. She turns away from her best friend and attends studiously to the speaker. She doubts he has done much work with women who were sexually abused.

"So you guys in the middle had the question about intimacy," says Evans. "What did you come up with? How about you?" and he points to a small gray-haired woman standing up in the back.

Mary and Karen swivel in their seat to listen to her.

She says with a deep, resonant voice, "I think it's pretty obvious. It's when you and your partner can be your true selves and be open with each other, and that both of you are able to respond with understanding and tenderness. It's not about romance; it's about having a best friend you can trust in the mess of everyday life. My partner and I call it love amidst the ruins. Being in love is nice, don't get me wrong, but living love is true intimacy."

The audience breaks into applause.

"Sounds good to me," says Jack, "but how does it work when your partner needs to share his honest and true feelings of frustration or disappointment with you?"

"Now that's getting a little personal and, by the way, my partner is a she and not a he."

"I'm sorry. It was a stupid assumption. I should. . . . "

"Don't go there," she says strongly. "It happens all the time. I don't want to deal with your heterosexualism. You deal with it."

Mary and Karen both laugh along with the rest of the audience at the presenter getting nailed. Jack ducks behind the podium and calls out "Incoming." Then he stands up and says, "Well said and fair enough. What were you going to say about how you and she manage conflict?"

"Honestly, if you really want to know, we just muddle through. In a funny way we both know that we're not exactly the easiest people in the world. Sometimes I just have to look in the mirror and say to myself, 'Honey, just remember you're no prize either.' So we cut each other some slack. That's all. Nobody says this is easy. But stuff does blow over. Besides, most of the time I'm able to convince her she's in the wrong."

"That sounds like a neat trick. Is your partner here? Let me ask her. Is it true she's able to make you think it's mostly your fault?"

A woman considerably younger than the first stands up too and says with a coy toss of the head, "Well, it certainly works better if I let her think she's right all the time."

The audience applauds.

"Thanks to both of you. And who else has some thoughts about intimacy?"

One of the guys pipes up, "Well, I don't know if this counts or not. But I was in New York on 9/11, and two days after, I went down to ground zero. There were all these people milling about in almost total silence. A crush of people: all kinds, black–white, old–young, every ethnicity, and they all had a look of awe and horror on their face."

"I worked my way to the front of the police barricade. I was standing there next to this black guy. He was holding a gold-framed picture of a girl in a white prom dress. He sees me looking. His eyes are filled with tears. My eyes well up. We look at each other for a long time. And then he nods and walks away." He pauses as he chokes back tears. "Weird as it may sound, it was one of the most intimate moments of my life."

The room is silent.

Mary watches Evans. Clearly, he doesn't know what to say. The silence feels right to her. Jason was in Manhattan on 9/11. He saw the second tower come down. He still refuses to talk about it.

Finally, Evans says quietly. "Let's let this moment of silence be for all of those who have gone and for the fathers and mothers, sisters and brothers, lovers and friends that were left behind."

Everyone bows their heads.

*　　*　　*

Karen wrestles a chunk of a cheesesteak into her mouth while Mary picks at her salad.

"So what's happening with Jason?" asks Karen, her mouth full. "Is he going to try and go back next semester?"

Mary's chest tightens. She reaches for the little pitcher of dressing on the side and splashes it all over her salad. "We don't know what's happening with him. We're trying to get him into some kind of therapy. Frank's too damn easy on the kid. Jason needs more of the tough than the love right now, but I'm always coming across like the Wicked Witch of the West. I don't know, I really don't know."

Karen leans across the table. "You know, if you don't mind me being a bit of a buttinsky, it sounds like you guys should consider some family therapy."

"I know, but I can't imagine how I could drag both of them in there. Besides, I know everybody around."

135

"Well, ask Evans. He used to work in Philly, and maybe he still has some good contacts."

"Karen, you're too much. I'm not about to go up to a presenter, a complete stranger, and ask for a referral."

*　　*　　*

Jack stretches out on a sofa that's tucked away in a corner of the lobby. The morning wasn't too bad, and he handled the gaffe with the lesbian okay. The guy who talked about 9/11 touched everyone. Wonder what my cabbie, Lou, would say if he had been there? What if Skipper had been there? The old man had never come to one of his trainings, even when Jack was in Scottsdale, five miles from his dad's house. "A very important golf game" had been the excuse at the time. The clench of the old ache surprises him. His dad didn't come to Little League either. He was always doing "very important business," his mother would say. If he pushed harder, she'd trot out the well-worn excuse about how Skipper lost his dad in World War I and really didn't know about how to father well—that he did the best he could.

Jack wonders what his dad would think if he came to one of his trainings. Would he have been impressed, maybe even proud?

Ann pops into his head. What would she have thought of the Great Jack Evans Show?

Jack closes his eyes and drifts off, hoping to get a little rest before the afternoon performance.

*　　*　　*

Mary likes the afternoon session better than the morning. The guy seems to be less caught up in being an entertainer and seems to know his stuff about sexual abuse. However, she couldn't help shaking her head when he told about having one survivor defuse her trauma trigger by tying a pink satin bow around her husband's penis. It's pretty hard to imagine any man going along with that idea.

"I'm not tying a frigging bow around my thing," Frank would say.

Luckily, she only had to run the typical girl's gauntlet, like having her bra snapped in sixth grade, Johnny Diregorio waving his thing at her on the bus, the nuns drilling the fear of God into her with their ominous warnings like "Once you give it away, you can never get it back," and that bulldog Physical Education instructor who said, "Remember, girls, don't linger when you are washing yourselves. Baths are for cleanliness." The thought of Sister Margaret's concern about "lingering" in the bath makes her smile. Nobody even knew what the Sister was talking about back then.

"Now," says Evans, "I want us to shift gears from our clients' grief and consider our own. We all carry some deep loss. I remember a line from a movie I saw, 'People die, relationships don't.' "

Mary snaps out of her reverie. He's going on about forgiveness and amends in their personal lives and then, suddenly, he's asking them all to write a note to someone right now.

"I'm not doing that," Mary whispers to Karen.

"Oh, go ahead. Everyone else is. He's doing it too."

Mary looks at her lined notebook. It looks like a final exam blue book. She doesn't feel like writing anything, but she's always done what she's been told. Maybe she should write Frank a letter of apology about their sex life. No! What if they have it to read to each other? She begins to doodle on the page. Everyone around her seems so studiously engaged. Then she knows.

Dear Jason,

I remember how bad I used to feel if I didn't get an A on everything. I was so afraid of making mistakes. And ever since you had trouble learning to read and write in first grade, I was always on your back. What was it like for you not being able to concentrate and just sitting doodling when everyone else was working hard?

Mary puts down her pen and reaches for the tissues in her purse. She daubs at her eyes so as not to make a mess of her mascara. Karen is still writing furiously away. She bends back to the page.

*I don't know why I didn't get you tested. It just seemed
like you didn't care about doing well. I thought you needed
more discipline. But all my nagging hasn't done the slightest
bit of good. Maybe it was the biggest mistake I ever made.
And now I don't know what to do. I love you and I'm so
sorry.*

Mom

She wipes her eyes again, and Karen reaches over and pats her
knee. Mary shakes her head and smiles back at Karen.

"Well, that was tougher than I expected," says Dr. Evans. "Over
the years, I've done this exercise with a lot of audiences and I feel
like it's unfair to spring it on you unless I do it alongside you without any preplanning. What I wrote surprised me but I would like to
share it with you, and I hope some of you might be willing to read
what you wrote, too."

"Not on your life," whispers Mary, and gets an elbow to the ribs
from Karen.

She looks at Evans putting on his reading glasses and is
voyeuristically intrigued.

"Dear . . . " Evans looks up at the audience. It's clear that's he's
trying to compose himself.

"Let me explain first, this is a letter to an old client of mine who
recently committed suicide. She actually wrote me a suicide note,
and I need to reach out to her husband and her children, which I
haven't done yet. I think this letter is a step. Obviously I'm not going
to mention her name. So here goes."

*I was so sorry and so sad to get your note. I had allowed
myself to believe that no news was good news. I know that you
fought courageously all through these years and that you did the
best you could to be a good mom to your kids and keep the
demons of your illness at bay.*

*I will reach out to them and help them as best I can. And, of
course, I. . . .*

He looks away and puts his hand over his eyes. "I'm sorry, I didn't expect this to be so hard." He swipes at his eyes with his sleeve. "Let me just finish. All of us face the risk of losing a client to suicide everyday. I'm reading this for her, and for me and each of you who does this sometimes godforsaken lonely job. Sorry." He smiles at the audience. "That seems a little over the top. Here's the end."

I know that I made mistakes and our work was really never the same for you after the Intervention and, well, there's so much to say and actually really nothing at all except I will remember you always. I am so sorry that you needed to do this.

With caring,

Jack

Mary reaches again for her tissues. She's moved in spite of herself. She remembers her own chronic fear of losing one of her patients. Then her stomach clenches so hard she almost gasps. It's Jason. This could be him. She feels like racing home to make sure he's okay.

Karen leans over and whispers, "Are you all right?"

Mary nods quickly despite her hands being clenched into tight fists in her lap.

"Is there anyone else who might be willing to share what they wrote?" Evans asks the audience. People shift around in their seats. There's an uncomfortable silence.

"Suddenly, I can't even make eye contact with you guys," teases Evans, "Please don't leave me hanging out to dry here."

A hand in the back is raised, and a small, wiry Chinese man gets up. The seeing-eye dog next to him pricks up his ears.

The audience swings around to see him.

The man awkwardly swings his head from one side to the other as if he is looking at the audience and then says, "It's, well, I don't write except inside my own head. Before I became blind I used to love to write. But, anyway, I do have a letter in my mind. Is that okay?"

"It's okay. It really is," says Evans.

Mary is almost holding her breath. It's hard to believe the man will do it.

"Well," he begins, "it's kind of one of those amends letters. It's for my three children. I say to them that I am so sorry that I am their father and that I cannot see them. I can't see them smile. And I can't play simple games with them, like catch with my sons, or enjoy my daughter's drawings. My wife says she has a lot of talent, you know. And I want so much for them to know how much I love them and how hard it is sometimes for them to always have to be explaining about having a blind dad who can't do many things that other dads can do. I don't know. I just want them to know that I see them with all my heart. That's all."

There is a long hush as the man finds his seat. Then Mary, Karen, everyone, even Evans, burst into applause. The man stands up and bows his head to everyone, gives a big smile, and then waves. The dog jumps up alertly. He wags his tail.

Evans says softly, "I'm sure your children feel your love and feel fully known by you."

Mary leans toward Karen and smiles in spite of herself. "Why didn't you tell me this was going to be a damn encounter group?"

Karen smiles back at her with tears in her eyes. "Who knew?"

*   *   *

Jack looks at the towering cumulonimbus clouds that they're headed toward and wonders whether the plane will be delayed by the thunderstorms. There's a spattering of raindrops on the cab windshield as they wait at a red light. He's annoyed that they might not make the plane and already gnawing over the day, feeling like reading the note to Ann was inappropriate. But then the blind guy just blew everyone away. The audience was deeply responsive, and isn't that really the point? But still, Jack worries.

"So, where are you headed?" interrupts the young black man driving the cab. He has a fine English accent and is wearing a multicolored dashiki reminiscent of the kind Jack wore in the 1960s.

"Back to Boston," replies Jack. He looks at the cabbie's picture and sees that he's riding with the American Cab Company again, and this time his driver is Ahmed Massariah.

"Boston is a good place. Many, many students. But so serious."

"What do you mean?"

A horn honks behind them and Ahmed steps on the gas. He smiles back at Jack with a broad grin. "You really want to know what it is that I think?

"Sure," says Jack, smiling back.

"Well, the problem is like all you Americans, they are so busy getting ahead they don't know where they are. You people have so much and nobody's happy. People just go round working hard, buying everything, and not having any fun."

"How do you know this?"

"Eyes."

"What?"

"None of your people have smiles in their eyes. They are too busy. Their eyes are always looking about. Always wanting something more. Not like in my country."

"So where are you from?" says Jack, wondering if Ahmed would think his eyes are smiling.

"Ethiopia."

"And are your people happy?"

Ahmed turns around in the cab and says with a big grin, "Yes. Absolutely."

"How does that work? I mean, hasn't there been a terrible civil war going on for years?" Jack wonders if his knowledge of African current events is in order. He's not sure whether it's Yemen or Ethiopia that's having the civil war.

"You name it, we got it. War, pestilence, poverty, starvation, corruption. Everything."

"So, listen, Ahmed. May I call you that?"

"Sure, man, what do they call you?

"Jack, This is . . "

"It's a pleasure to be meeting you, Mr. Jack."

"Likewise. Anyway, what you're saying is really interesting. With all that stuff going on, how can your people be so happy?"

"Simple. It's people treating people like people."

"What?"

"Maybe I'm not so clear. Really it's two things. Family and religion. Back home we treat every one as family, so between the religious holidays and the birthdays and the funerals, there's always a party going on. We treat all strangers like they're friends and all things to do are for fun. We make everything fun. Even your Presidents. Some of the time, please don't take offense, we are having fun just talking about your presidents, like cowboy Bush and, how do you say, horny, that's it, yes, horny Bill."

Jack laughs. The traffic has slowed to a standstill. He glances at his watch.

"You want to hear a joke, Mr. Jack?

"Go for it, Mr. Ahmed."

"What do you call the Clinton time, you know what I mean, that administration?"

"Beats me."

"Sex between the Bushes."

Jack bursts out laughing. It was hard to imagine how Ahmed and Lou Abrizzi work for the same cab company.

They inch up next to the car that's stalled and blocking the traffic. The woman in the teal business suit standing in front of the raised hood looks familiar. He can't figure where he's seen her before. Just as they are about to pick up speed, Jack says, "Ahmed, pull over, will ya?"

*   *   *

Mary is bent over her steaming engine, and she's steaming. Her radiator has broken and AAA said it will take an hour. And it's about to rain like hell. She looks back at the line of stuck commuters and shrinks with guilt about making them all late. She peers intently back under the hood.

"Hey, weren't you in my workshop today?"

Mary turns around and there's Dr. Evans, standing next to her, smiling. She's speechless.

"Come on. I'll give you a ride to a gas station. My cab's right here." He points to Ahmed, who's standing by the cab in the breakdown lane just behind him.

"No, it's really okay. I've already called AAA. But thanks, I mean, you know, for stopping."

"Sure. To tell the truth, I probably wouldn't have except I remembered you from today. It's easy to talk about being a supportive community. But I don't always practice what I preach."

"Well, who does?" Mary smiles, pleased he stopped. Then she hesitates, "Um, listen, I'm sorry to bother you, but my friend said you might know some really good family therapists and, well, I'm a therapist and I shouldn't be unable to manage my own child, but I, uh, need a referral. I mean, my son, we need to get some help."

"Well, I've got just the person for you. He's Dr. John Pappenow and he's great with boys and their families."

"I really appreciate this."

"No problem. Is this worry about your son what you wrote about, you know, in the workshop?"

Mary begins to tear up and turns away.

"I'm sorry. I mean here we are standing in the middle of a traffic jam and. . . . "

"It's okay," Mary interrupts him. "I wrote to him. I apologized. I feel so bad about how hard I was on him, and I don't know if he's going to be okay."

"That's rough. I think the worst thing on the planet is realizing that sometimes we've been hurtful to our kids. I feel that way about my daughter. I actually am thinking about going back into therapy myself over it. Listen, may I suggest something?"

"Yes." She looks him straight in the eye.

"Well, this is probably going to sound a little hokey, but, hey, I guess you already know that about me," he says with a slight shrug.

"Sometime, while he's lying in bed sound asleep and you can see him, just as he is, just a big version of the little boy he used to be, and no matter what kind of mess he's making of his life and how frustrated you might be with him, read him what you wrote."

"I think I ought to just read it to him when he's awake," Mary counters.

"Well, maybe. You certainly know better than I do," Jack says with a smile, and sticks out his hand. "Anyway, I've got to run."

Mary impulsively step toward him and gives him a big hug. "Thank you," she whispers.

They turn and see Ahmed leaning against the side of his cab. He's grinning at them and giving them a thumbs up.

QUESTIONS FOR DISCUSSION

1. Do you sometimes feel isolated as a clinician? How do you get support and your sense of community?
2. Ahmed describes the alienation that he sees in American culture. What's your experience of American culture? What do you think are the bonds that create community?
3. Jack's workshop exercise was emotionally intense for the audience and for Jack. Was it appropriate for him to share his letter to Ann and to encourage other participants to share their letters? How do you feel about teachers in the field being vulnerable and acknowledging that they make mistakes?
4. Jack chose being a therapist as a way of staying true to his commitment to service and caring, and yet he feels sometimes like he's a "fraud" or a "rent-a-friend." Have you ever had feelings like that? Why? What have you done about them?

5. Is Mary experiencing some vicarious traumatization in her work with sexual abuse survivors, and how might it affect her fears about her son?
6. Mary is uncomfortable asking for help. Have you ever felt that because you're a clinician you shouldn't need help? What have you done about it?

INTO THE
WILD BLUE

The sandpipers scuttled on delicate toothpick legs, chasing the receding waves. Hurriedly, they pecked at invisible life in the wet sand. As each new wave crashed in, they rushed back up the beach like toddlers afraid of the water.

The wind was coming off the sea. The sun was warm despite the late summer chill in the air. Not quite sunbathing weather. The beach was nearly deserted except for the three generations of the Evans family sitting in a row.

It was the last day of vacation on the Vineyard, and Alex had insisted on one last visit to the beach before they loaded up the car. Her father and granddad had come along too. Skipper hated the beach, but he doted on his youngest granddaughter. He liked her tough, no-nonsense style and already missed her as he contemplated her departure for college. She was disappearing into adulthood right before his eyes. It had been a long time since she climbed on his lap and said, "Grand, tell me a story." Despite having grumped about it's being much too cold for the beach, the difficulties of walking on sand, and the greasiness of suntan lotion, he was content to steal some time alone with Alex and Jack, away from the endless waves of chatter that dominated the annual gathering of his clan.

Despite being 91, Skipper still looked indomitable. His weather-beaten lines and splotches of brown age spots didn't diminish the clarity of his Gulf Stream blue eyes. He was staring out to sea the same way he did from the bridge of his beloved destroyer, the *USS Carolina*. Being by the water always reminded Skipper of the comfortable rhythms of his life at sea. It was a damn sight easier out there being Captain John Evans than navigating through the world of retirement, grandparenting, and golf had been. He accepted the duties of being the patriarch of this mélange of children, spouses, and grandchildren, but the physical realities of old age were an assault on his dignity. He couldn't do much anymore. Just walking was a bitch. He had a barrel chest and big belly perched on thin, stalk-like legs, and he was so damn pigeon-toed that it made each step a balancing act, and now he could barely move without being out of breath. But he wouldn't accept help and dismissed his wife's insistence that he use a cane as the nattering of an old woman.

Alex sat to the left of her Dad and Skipper and basted herself with suntan lotion. She was glad she'd brought a book. Her father might start trying to "talk," and all she wanted to do was stop time. She looked out at the deserted beach. Ever since she was little, she'd always been the last one to be dragged out of the water at the end of the day.

"Alex, you are turning as blue as ocean, it's time to go," her father would say.

"I'm not cold," she'd sputter, despite pulling the beach towel tightly around her and shivering all over.

"I'm getting cold just looking at you." Then he swooped her up and swung her over his shoulder.

"Please, please," she'd beg, and he'd always let her weasel another 10 minutes in the water.

She should be back at the house helping her mom and Megan with the packing, but she couldn't face it. The minute they got home she'd have to start getting ready for college, and she really wasn't ready to deal with it, or anything else for that matter. She shivered.

Jack had hoped to have a little time alone with Alex at the beach and had gently tried to discourage Skipper from coming. "Don't bother with it, Dad. We'll only be down there for less than an hour and you know the walk may be a little much."

"I'll decide how much walking is too much for me, thank you, Doctor. You're beginning to sound more like your mother every day."

" I'll take that as a compliment."

"You would."

"Stop it, you two. Let's just go to the beach," Alex silenced them.

Jack glanced over at Alex in her turquoise bikini. She definitely had lost weight this summer. For the last couple of months she had been even more withdrawn and crabby than usual. Ellen joked that it was nature's way of helping parents let their children fly from the nest.

Jack looked at her profile. Her lips were pursed, jaw set, arms folded across her chest as if to she were wearing a "Do not trespass" sign. Jack always assumed that because he was a good therapist, he would be able to communicate well with his children. It had been easy with Megan, who exuberantly wanted to go over every micro-detail of her life with him. But Alex rarely talked. Even when she was little, she was too busy, doing elaborate jigsaw puzzles, collecting things, and playing games. Whether it was cards, Monopoly, or even chess, Alex was a ferocious competitor with the family. She loved beating Jack in particular. He stopped helping her win by the time she was eight. She didn't need it.

When she was still little, Jack was able to coax her into an occasional talking game. He invited her into his home office at the end of his day and she would pretend to be a client, and or she would sit in his leather chair and, with complete seriousness, be a therapist. Under the guise of pretending, the conversations were often startlingly direct, like when she was eight and challenged the whole idea of heaven as a fairy tale made up to comfort children but she wasn't afraid of dying, anyway. Another time she asked him if he loved her mother as much as he did the day they got married. Jack had stumbled around, muttering things about how love changes like the seasons, and she brusquely cut him off and pronounced that obviously nobody felt the same way all their life, and that's why she planned on having several different husbands, like Callie's mom. Or maybe marriage wouldn't be for her, anyway. Jack was taken aback by her practicality. Pity the poor boy who messes around with her, he thought.

Their communication had worsened since she started high school. Whenever he attempted more meaningful topics than curfews, cars, and allowance, he'd get back some variation of "Stop being such a shrink, Dad. Save it for your paying customers."

It saddened Jack to realize that he was better at talking with his clients than with his own daughter. He remembered Friday's session with Molly O'Leary. He had worked with the O'Leary family off and on for 11 years. Both Tom and Molly had grown up under the shadow of substance abuse. Tom had been active alcoholic for 20 years but was finally sober through AA, and now their son, Joe, had become a heroin addict.

Yesterday, Molly was furious with Joe and the whole situation. She read a poignant note that their seven-year-old grandson, Tommy, had written to his dad, begging him to get help.

She read it out loud and then said, "I wrote a pathetic letter like that to my father when I was the same age. I can't stand seeing that sweet little boy getting his heart broken, too."

Jack looked at the worn-out, distraught woman in front of him and caught a glimpse of the earnest little eight-year-old she had been. After he had her do some deep breathing meditation and make a mental list of all her negative feelings, he said, "If you could go back in time and just be with that little girl, knowing her the way you do, knowing everything about her, all her deepest fears, hopes, and dreams, what would you say to her?"

Molly paused and tears welled up in her eyes. "I'd tell her, no, first, I'd just hug her. That's all. I'd just hug her. Then I'd tell her she's okay and that it's not her fault."

Molly stopped crying and smiled. "I get what you're trying to do. You want me to do for little Tommy what I couldn't do for myself."

"Actually, Molly, I just wanted you to do it for you. But you could do it for Tommy, too. It's a good idea."

At the end of the hour, Molly thanked him and said, "Thanks, Doc, thanks for being there."

Jack glanced back over toward Alex. She leaned forward and looked past Jack toward Skipper, "Grand, what kind of shore birds are those down there? I've forgotten." She pointed toward the water's edge.

"Well, Peaches, those are sandpipers. Can you tell if they're spotted? I can't see from here."

"Yes, they have little brown spots and dark wings and backs."

"The spotted pipers are usually the ones we see here on the island. One year I did see some different ones. I wasn't sure whether they were actually pipers or some kind of plover. I think they were the solitary sandpiper."

Jack sighed. Skipper was always the expert, on any conceivable topic. Jack shrugged and let the two of them talk right through him. He looked out to sea at a sailboat laboring against the wind. It was rail down, bashing into the waves, and making very little way.

Skipper was in full form, as if he were still lecturing at the Naval Academy. "So you see, each species is assigned a scientific name which is made up of two parts, first the genus and then the species. Our spotted sandpiper is called *Actitis macularia.*"

"Dad," Jack said, "she just wanted to know what kind of bird it was. You're beginning to sound like Roger Tory Peterson himself." Jack hoped this was a light shot across the old man's bow.

"Well, my boy, it's nice to have a child who will listen to an old man," harrumphed his father.

Jack bit his tongue. He hadn't come to the beach to bicker with his father. They did that enough already. Jack had once idolized his old man, and he hungered for his approval. But no matter what Jack did, there was always more yardage to be gained or a better grade to be had. "Our best today, better tomorrow" was Skipper's favorite motto.

Then the Vietnam War hit. Skipper was finished with active duty and teaching at the Academy. Jack's two older brothers were over there, Frank in the Marines and Jim in the Navy. Jack was a freshman in college, into sex, drugs, and rock and roll. Then he joined the peace movement. Jack in his hippie uniform and Skipper in his pressed khaki could barely be in the same room together. Jack remembered attacking the old man as if he were Lyndon Johnson himself. They fought constantly while his mom fluttered between them. Finally they just didn't talk about the war.

After his dad sold Shady Hill and moved to Scottsdale, their conflict had died down. Their last big fight was about the old homestead. First his dad tried to get one of his older brothers to move back East to take over the farm. When that didn't work, he pushed Jack hard to buy it, offering it at $200,000 below market price. Jack had insisted it was too big and needed to much upkeep for him and Ellen to manage. "But it's been in the family for 131 years. My people are buried there," he'd said, sounding both plaintive and accusatory. Jack felt pulled hard, but stood his ground.

Now the bickering between them felt like the dying embers of those years. Without the occasional spark, all they ever talked about was sports, the stock market, or the kids. Occasionally Jack succumbed to sending his dad articles he wrote or brochures of workshops, despite getting back only crumbs of approval like "So Jack, it sounds like you're becoming a big fish in that pond of yours."

Jack glanced over at his father. The visor and aviator sunglasses mostly hid his face. Skipper had finished his lecture, and Jack couldn't tell if he was awake or asleep. He looked old. Jack wondered about how Skipper felt about being old and facing death. There was so much they'd never talked about, like the war in the South Pacific or even stuff about Skipper's childhood and his growing up without a dad.

Soon the old man would be gone.

Jack turned back to Alex, her face buried in her book. He reached over and tapped her shoulder. "Hey, did you hear back from your roommate yet?"

"No."

"Are you going to try her again?"

"Dad, I already tried. If she wants to talk, fine. If not, I'll be meeting her soon enough." She disappeared back into her book.

Jack looked back out to sea. The sailboat was barely making

progress. Must be a strong contrary current out there. The late afternoon sun slanted over the water, and there was a big patch of glittering gold sprinkled over the blue. He tried to let the sparkling beauty soothe him. He sat up and reached for his polo shirt. There was a chill in the sea breeze.

He thought back to how well the session had ended with Molly O'Leary. She had found that little guided visualization exercise very useful.

Maybe he needed to practice a little of what he preached. So far he'd found this jaunt to the beach agitating. Jack closed his eyes and began meditating—just following the rise and fall of his chest, the in breath and the out breath. He began to settle down. Work with clients was a whole lot easier than trying to relate to his family. At least when he was the shrink, he knew what his job was. Jack felt so distant from Alex, and she was leaving for Stanford the day after tomorrow. He was still hurt that she had spurned his offer to go out with her on the plane and help her move in. "Come on, Dad, kids nowadays don't show up with a parent in tow."

Jack opened his eyes and looked at the two of them: Alex engrossed in her book, her hair blowing across her face, Skipper with his head down on his chest. They seemed miles away. Jack remembered how intimately connected he felt with Molly O'Leary when he guided her through the exercise. What if he asked Skipper and Alex to do it? Of course, they'd make fun of the idea. But maybe he ought ask them to do it anyway, just as a favor to him, if nothing else.

Suddenly he remembered his encounter with Ahmed, and his impulsive decision to stop for the woman by the side of the road. That worked out. Life's short. What did he have to lose? He'd rather mix it up with them somehow than sit there in a row, three silent bumps on a beach.

"Hey, you two, how about us doing something different? I'd really like to get some feedback from you two about this guided imagery exercise I've been doing with my clients to see what you think of it. It will only take a few minutes."

"Dad," groaned Alex, "why do you have wreck a perfectly good afternoon with some dumb therapy exercise?"

"The girl's got a point," chimed in Skipper.

Normally, Jack would accept their rebuff with a self-deprecatory joke. But he was determined.

"Listen, humor me a bit. It'll only take a few minutes and you don't have to talk about what you feel if you don't want to. Let me explain how it works. . . . "

"Dad, I'd rather do the dumb thing than hear a lecture about it." She glanced over at Skipper and said with a wink, "Sometimes, it is better just to humor him, Grand."

"Don't I know it."

"We'll do it, Dad, if you really mean we don't have to talk about it. Sounds like, maybe, you're the one that needs it."

"All right, all right, maybe I do. I know it sounds hokey, but just hang in there. We'll all do it together. The first part is simple. Basic meditation. Just sit back. Get comfortable and close your eyes. Notice your experience of breathing, the air coming in and out, the rise and fall of your chest."

Jack looked from one to the other. Alex sat up straight in her beach chair with her legs folded in the lotus position and her left hand over her right in her lap. She had learned some basic meditation in school. Skipper hadn't moved at all, and Jack couldn't even tell if he had closed his eyes. What the hell, he can do it any way he wants.

"Just focus on your breathing, and when other thoughts come into your head let them float on by as if they were just clouds passing through the sky or the waves rolling up the beach."

Jack saw Alex shake her head ever so slightly and knew he was talking too much. He focused on his own breath. He felt the wind on his face and heard the rolling sound of the surf. His busy brain settled down.

At the end of a couple of minutes, Jack said softly, "Now, we're just going to keep breathing and let our minds open to all the negative feelings we might have. Anything you feel sad, mad, or, bad about—anything that's worrying you. Just list all those feelings one at a time as you keep on breathing, one breath at a time.

So the Evans family sat, eyes closed, by the water's edge.

When Jack started in with his "just breathe in and breathe out" bit, Skipper shook his head. And now he was supposed to be thinking negative thoughts? Damn, it was bad enough being on the beach without having to do this touchy-feely stuff. He should be back there getting people organized because the whole airport scene was such a hassle after the 9/11 mess. Don't get me started, he thought. This Bush kid is so out in left field without a paddle and he struts around like a runt gamecock thinking it's his cock-a-doodle-do that's bringing the sun up. His Iraq saber rattling was bullshit. Where the hell was the military? Why couldn't the Joint Chiefs rein him in? There really hadn't been a decent leader since Eisenhower. Ike wouldn't have tied the military's hands behind their back in Vietnam.

Skipper shifted his weight. Thinking of Vietnam brought up his vivid memories of Jack and his stupid dirty long blond hair and his Army surplus jacket. How often he would explode at the dinner table because Jack just didn't make any sense and then Jack would walk out and he'd be left with his wife and daughter in tears, acting like it was all his fault. He remembered how ashamed he'd been of Jack, and how proud of his other two sons who were over there.

But it did change when Jack became 1A and said that he was prepared to go to jail rather than run for Canada. He said it was his patriotic duty to be willing to pay the price for his position. Skipper felt both afraid for his boy's safety and some real pride in his guts. Finally he was acting like a man. Skipper never argued about the war again with Jack. He wondered if he had ever told Jack that he respected his decision. Or even that by the time of Nixon's Cambodian invasion, he agreed with him. Wasn't at all like World War II, when everyone knew who were the bad guys.

Skipper's mind flashed back to being on board the USS Carolina, his ship. The fleet was steaming toward Midway Island with rumors there was going to be some major action somewhere up ahead. Skipper couldn't sleep. He was prowling the bridge like a caged tiger. There was no moon and they were blacked out, so the bridge was completely dark. He stuck his head outside and listened to the dull rumble of the diesels and watched the silvery splash of the bow wave as his ship sliced through black water. He was scared witless. Just as afraid as he used to be when he was little. Nothing at the Naval Academy or the countless hours of drills and exercises had prepared him for feeling like this. He always assumed he would be cool, calm, and collected going into action. And here he was, the commander of a destroyer with 270 men depending on him, and he felt like he would shit his pants. It wasn't that he was afraid of dying. No, he was more afraid he'd lose it in front of his men or make a mistake that would get some of his guys killed or cost him his ship. What the hell was he doing commanding this ship, anyway? He'd been made the youngest commander in the fleet. He felt like a complete fraud.

"Damn this stupid therapist shit," he muttered and his eyes snapped open and he looked over at Jack, who was still meditating. I'm way too old to be remembering stuff like that. He hadn't thought about that night for 58 years. He could still smell the sea, see the bow wave, feel the stab of fear in his belly. Funny how you can remember things clear as a bell from back then, but what about the last 20 years? He suddenly remembered being in the barn with his dad before he died in World War I. Phew. That was more than 80 years ago.

Then he heard himself think, don't worry Skip, it won't be long. You're almost done.

*   *   *

Alex settled into the breathing easily, but she couldn't believe her father had pushed them to do this. Grand must be going out of his mind! Dad and his stupid shrink things, but she felt sorry for him after being mean to him all summer. Still, he should understand how it is between kids and their dads. After all, he was a shrink. None of her friends talked anywhere near as much to their fathers as she did. Why was he always guilt tripping her?

She slumped a little in her chair. The hell with the meditation posture. She definitely wasn't going to make a list of everything that made her feel bad. Thank God she was finally starting school and getting away from everything.

Then it all came back. She had tried to blot out it out of her mind all summer. The June prom. Nobody knew how excited she'd been that Jamie Ellison had asked her. She'd had a secret crush on him since freshman year. And it started so well, the perfect dress, a cream-colored strapless just the right length, the picture session, the limo, the dinner at La Nuit. Everything was great until the drinking started. At the after-prom, everybody was sipping out of little flasks and she decided just this once to drink. The next thing she knew Jamie was coaxing her into going up to his buddies' hotel room. The rest was all a blur of smells, sweat, weight, and hurt. Did she try to push him away? Say no? She couldn't remember anything except lurching to the bathroom afterward and puking her guts out and cleaning up the blood from down there. When she came back to the bedroom, there he was lying naked on the bed showing off everything, smoking a cigarette, a big smirk on his face. She wanted to smack that look right off him. But she had to get out of there. She didn't even ask him if he had used a rubber. She was such a damn idiot.

She couldn't bear to tell anyone, not even Callie. For 10 days she held her breath waiting for her period. Finally, when it came, she remembered the rush of relief, but her anger and shame stayed. Instead of being mad at Jamie, she was pissed at herself. She couldn't believe she'd been so stupid. She had always told her friends that she wasn't going to be dumb enough to give it away to some pawing adolescent boy. When she looked at herself in the mirror she felt like shredding her face with her nails.

The whole thing wrecked her summer; she completely shut down. All she did was her Buddy Dog job for the Humane Society, watch TV, and count the days until she could leave. Maybe then she'd get a clean start. Dad knew something was wrong. He kept probing at her about why she wasn't going out or seeing her friends. Once she might have actually wanted to talk to him. They could have played his stupid therapy game. But not now. Not about this.

Suddenly, Alex missed being little. She missed her daddy, the cuddling up next to him when he read her stories. He read her *The Secret Garden* start to finish when she was nine. She told him she was way too old for bedtime stories, but she loved it. The whole idea of getting on the plane next week by herself seemed utterly impossible. Why had she refused her dad's offer to come with her? Her mom couldn't, but Dad would have rearranged his schedule. Alex felt hopelessly pigheaded, stupid, and afraid.

*   *   *

Jack's breathing was ragged. He was embarrassed about imposing the exercise on the other two. Imagining how stupid they thought it was released a rush of self-loathing: His dad never respected him, thought his profession was for the birds, never forgave him for antiwar protests. Alex didn't respect him as either a dad or a shrink and had been avoiding him like the plague. Ellen reminded him several times to stop taking it so personally, that it wasn't really about him—advice that he had been giving parents for years. Now she's leaving for college and she didn't even want him to take her.

His mind flashed on holding Alex's hand at the bus stop when she was five years old, her first time getting on the school bus. He remembered her blond hair in braids, her furrowed brow, and the look of anxious determination. She had held onto his hand so tightly, but dropped it quickly as soon as the bus was in sight. He could see her stepping up into the yawning mouth of the yellow beast; she never looked back. He stood on the street and watched the bus slowly disappear. Here she was going again, and this time she didn't want to let him in, even a little. Why couldn't he help his own daughter, when he spent all his days helping other people with this same stuff? Was he just a fraud? He remembered those first days at boarding school, when it felt like he put on his personality just like he put on the school uniform every day, and why the hell did he still have all these feelings, despite having been in psychotherapy off and on for years?

Then he fell into a well of grief. He felt so sad for Alex. Despite her tough demeanor, she had plenty of insecurity, even shyness. He even felt a deep sadness for the old man next to him who was not far from setting off on his own journey. Home would be the sailor, home from the sea. Was the old man afraid of the pain and humiliation of dying? How would he take to the indignities of diapers, tubes, and patronizing nurses washing him like a baby?

Then Jack found himself picturing saying good-bye to both of them, and his eyes filled up. He felt tenderness and love for these two that went way beyond words.

He opened his eyes and looked over at them. Less than three minutes had gone by. Suddenly he realized that the part of the exercise he did with Molly O'Leary could just be needlessly emotional for all of them. He decided to make the last part of the exercise easier, a more soothing variation than what he had done with Molly.

"Now take a deep breath, hold it for a second and let it all the way out," Jack said softly. He told them to imagine being in a special place where they were completely comfortable, relaxed, and accepting of themselves just as they are. "It could be anywhere, on a mountainside, next to a brook, a favorite place you had as a child."

*   *   *

Jack was talking in his irritating soft voice and Skipper couldn't follow what he was getting at. He had a momentary flash of the utter contentment and exhaustion he felt lying in his bunk as the *Carolina* was steaming ENE toward Honolulu three days after VJ Day. He could almost feel the gentle roll of the ship. It would be good to get back to the farm. His head nodded.

*   *   *

Alex was relieved that this thing was almost over. She couldn't imagine what this place was supposed to be like. Then she saw herself on a path in the woods. Her mother and father were holding each hand and swinging her. She could see the flashing oranges and reds of the leaves, the canopy of deep blue sky. They were all laughing. She remembered her dad singing, on the upswing, "Up she goes, up into the wild blue yonder, into the sky."

*   *   *

Jack had done this exercise a lot and always imagined going to the side of a mountain stream, resting with his back against a tree and listening to the burbling rush of the water. But he couldn't get out of his negative thinking. God, he hoped that Alex or Skipper hadn't gotten stuck in it, too.

He surreptitiously looked at them. Skipper's head had fallen forward and his jaw was slack. For a second, Jack thought he was dead; no, his old man was just sleeping like a baby. On his other side, Alex looked peaceful. He could see the trace of a smile playing on her face. Maybe this wasn't such a bad idea after all.

He glanced at his watch, 3:20. The women back at the house would be annoyed if they didn't get back right away. So he said softly, "Now just take one more deep cleansing breath, hold it all the way in for a second, and then let it go all the way out."

Alex slowly opened her eyes and looked at him. Jack put his finger to his lips and gestured with his thumb toward Skipper, who was snoring lightly,

"So, what was that like for you?" Jack asked.

"It was okay, Dad, but you said we didn't have to talk about it, right?

"Yup," said Jack. "I ended up feeling a little dumb about pushing you guys to do it. We certainly don't have to talk about it. Besides, we've got to get back. Why don't you wake Skipper? He'll be nicer to you."

Alex smiled and went over to her grandfather's chaise lounge and whispered, "It's time, Grand. Places to go, things to do."

Skipper woke up with a startle, looked at both of them, and pronounced, "Well, that takes the cake. Do you put all your customers asleep like that? The second you opened your mouth I dropped like a stone. People pay you for this? What a racket."

"It's okay, Dad. If all you got out of it was a little snooze, then no harm done, right?

"You're the doctor."

"Well, we've got to get back. Let us give you a hand."

Jack stood on one side and Alex on the other. They both reached

159

out a hand. Skipper grabbed for Alex and ignored Jack. "One of you is plenty," he said as he lurched to his feet. "You walk ahead of me and I'll just put my hand on your shoulder."

Jack busied himself picking up the towels and chairs as his father and daughter started wobbling up the beach. Skipper swayed from side to side with each step, but Alex was slow and steady.

Jack caught up with them.

"So, do you think we hid out long enough for them to get the packing done?" chuckled Skipper.

"So that's what got you to the beach, Dad. I was wondering."

"Well, it is women's work after all."

"Grand!" said Alex with mock outrage.

""Sorry, Peaches. You have to forgive the babblings of an old man. I am aware that times have changed."

They all laughed.

Alex glanced at her father. "You know, Dad," she paused, "well, if you really wanted to, it would be all right for you to take me out there. I mean, I was thinking that I am going to need help with all the boxes and stuff."

She quickly glanced away.

Before he could catch himself, Jack said, "Oh, sweetie, that would have been great, but I have a full schedule already. Besides, at this late date, the airfare would be horrendous. I don't even know if I could get on the flight."

"Yeah, yeah, I know, don't explain." She shrugged and turned away.

Dammit, Jack thought.

His father stopped and turned back to Jack. "You know what, son. You are a perfect horse's ass. Change your damn schedule, book the damn flight, and I damn well will pay for it. And for godsake, get your priorities straight."

Jack and Alex stopped in their tracks and stared at the old man.

"Aye, aye, Skipper," said Jack with a big grin. He squared his shoulders and saluted his father. The old man was right, but he'd be damned if he let him pay for it. They'd settle that later.

"And that, my boy, is a piss-poor civilian salute if I ever saw one."

QUESTIONS FOR DISCUSSION

1. Jack, Alex, and Skipper are each alone and troubled. They have difficulty talking intimately with each other. Do you recognize this kind of isolation and lack of communication in your own family? What do you do to bridge the gap? What works?
2. Jack was able to have intimate communication with his client, Molly, and yet is feeling inhibited with his father and his daughter. How does your being a clinician either enhance or harm your communication with your own family?
3. Alex has been devastated by being date raped and has been unable to tell any one. Date rape is very common and rarely acknowledged. Do you know either a client, friend, or family member who has had this experience? What do you think date rape does to an individual, and what do you think might help?
4. Skipper is facing the inevitability of his death, and he and Jack have never talked about it. How do you think people come to terms with their mortality?
5. Should Jack be the one to open up the issue or should he wait for Skipper to broach the subject? What would you do with your own aging parent?
6. There seems to be some reconnection between the three at the end. Did Jack's imposing his exercise on them actually work, or was it just serendipity?

2004

Not Exactly
a Chocolate Soufflé

I

Jack was frozen to his desk chair. Ellen was furious that he wasn't coming upstairs, but he'd be damned if he'd be the one to make the peace. He flipped through his appointment book looking at the next day's lineup and wondered what his couples would think if they saw this stupid, stubborn juvenile fight they were having. They hadn't had a fight like this in years. If their kids were still home they'd probably be reduced to talking through them, as in "Would you ask your mother to pass the salt?" Thirty-six years of marriages, two grown daughters, a good solid life, and he felt cold and angry in a way he hadn't in a long while. He always used to refer to these feelings melodramatically as his "dead man's mood." Ellen would dismissively call him "a sour puss." That would just piss him off even more.

It was like their early years, when everything he did was wrong. "Jack, there's place for everything and everything has its place," Ellen would say, holding up his razor at the sink, opening the cabinet, and demonstrating where to put it. Most of the time, he'd just smile and promise to try harder. If he tried to teasing like "Thank you honey, I never would have guessed that the razor should go up there," Ellen would get furious and stay that way until he made a groveling apology.

Thoughts about those early days made Jack cringe. It wasn't really Ellen's fault. He'd been so passive–aggressive back then. Always playing the nice guy while pretty much just taking her for granted. He had thrown himself into work and graduate school while she was bored at her part-time paralegal job and by being a housewife. Jack was enthralled with being a therapist. He worked 50 hours a week at the treatment center, plus all weekend on his dissertation.

He remembered one night when he got home late as usual, Ellen greeted him with "You care so much about all your drug-fiend criminal clients in that treatment center of yours, but you come home and you're just too, too tired to be with me."

Jack was speechless. She was right. At least at the treatment center, even the junkies who knew he was a just-out-of-school beginner cut him more slack than Ellen. He said, "You know, honey, I think you need more to do than have me as your makeover project. You've got a find something else to fuss about. You're kind of like a thermonuclear power plant hooked up to run a sewing machine."

She ran into the bedroom and cried the rest of the night. He felt like such shitball. He spent the night on the sofa. He was 22 years old. Six months married.

And now I'm almost 60, he thought, and having the same old feelings. Jack thought about his old journal that he had carefully hidden when Megan and Alex were little. He had stuck it inside some case folders way back in his filing cabinet. You never know. He remembered the thrilling shock of coming across the pornography in Skipper's sock drawer. Skipper would have killed him if he had known.

It was strange having the old man gone. All his life, Skipper had loomed over him like a towering thundercloud. Now he was gone. Not with a bang, not with a whimper, just gone: a message from his brother on the answering machine. "Jack. This is Frank. Skipper died in his sleep last night. Mom's okay. It was quick, just the way the old man would have wanted it."

And so that's a life. That's it. Jack's anger began to melt into sadness. His father had died a year ago, but Jack hadn't felt any real grief yet. Any feelings at all. Ellen had encouraged him to go back to see Beth. At some point he knew he would. He just wasn't ready to open that particular can of worms. Besides, it seemed like there ought to be a statue of limitations on childhood issues. Did he really need to go back over the ways in which his father wasn't there for him?

In the mood he was in, he didn't want to think about the old man. He dug out the 30-year-old journal and opened it. The last time he had read through it, he had felt riddled with shame. He had been so hurtful to Ellen back then. He didn't know what to expect this time. He was curious.

Jack's reading glasses slipped down his nose as he bent over the faded lines.

4/1/72. The lump in my bed is crying. I should be comforting her with soft, soothing "I'm sorrys" (that always works eventually), but I can't anymore. That well is bone dry. So I'm writing this instead. I've got to go soon. I'm wrecking both of us. My hate flicks at the air like the tongue of an adder when it's coiled and ready.

Nice literary metaphor, Jack. Are we trying to be a writer again? How droll. Using our pain for raw material? Creative Writing 101?

Christ! I'm just so pissed off. And she's still lying there accusing me with her sobbing. I hate that she gets to self-righteously blame me for everything even though it is mostly my fault. I don't give a flying fuck whose fault it is, I just have to get out of here. It's definitely April Fool's day.

4/15/72. Allston is the armpit of Boston. If this damn therapeutic separation is designed to teach me that the grass isn't greener, well, Allston's the right place for me to rent a room. And what a pit this is. It has the proverbial naked light bulb swinging over my bed. Of course, I couldn't spend our money on something decent. After all, I'm evil incarnate.

Ellen seems to be making a rather remarkable recovery. She was as cool as a cucumber or any other vegetable as we negotiated with Harney the funereal details. I don't know what's worse, her volcanic anger or her arctic chill. I can't stand the thought of what she sees when she looks at me.

Meanwhile Harney was relentlessly upbeat about this separation deal: a step toward saving our marriage. Right.

Robin is probably waiting for me. I don't know why I haven't gone over there. She'd be all over me. She's really into it. I've never been with a woman like her. I wish Ellen were more like that. But I can't deal with Robin tonight. Ever since I moved out, she's started the "what about us?" conversation. Talk about out of the frying pan and into the fire. I told her from the beginning that I was just an immature asshole. I loved Ellen, I wanted to work out the marriage and caveat emptor. "I'm damaged goods," I said. She just smiled and shushed me with her index finger to my lips. She whispered, "It's okay, we'll sing in the sunshine, we'll laugh everyday." Right. You, me, and Dusty Springfield.

4/21/72. Sweet Pea is dead. My whole therapy group was blown away. Apparently, he crossed over to the wrong side of Columbus Ave. Dragon's turf. Why wasn't he paying attention? He knew they had a price on him. Despite his innocent baby face and aw-shucks style, everyone knew he was the warlord of the "Dead Men." Dammit. He'd really been making progress. Last week in therapy, he broke down when he talked about stepping in front of his mother to take his father's drunken punches. He sobbed in Melvin's arms like a little boy.

Fuck! We never should have let him go out on pass. But he'd been doing so well, he'd earned it.

Jack looked up from the page. He remembered Sweet Pea. That kid was going to make it. Jack thought about his old group. What a motley crew of rapists, junkies, gang members, and murderers. In one 12-hour marathon session they'd really gotten close, so he asked them to come up with a name for themselves. They did. They even had it engraved on a beer mug that they gave him: "Endeavorers for a New Life." Most of the guys had ended up dead or back in prison. But not Melvin Johnson—he'd become a successful community leader in Roxbury. Jack had run into him at a fund-raiser just five years ago. Does he remember holding Sweet Pea? Jack wondered.

Jack picked up the journal again.

4/29/72. I can't sleep. God, I wish Ellen were here. What have I done? Robin and I don't belong together. What am I doing?

Jack smiled at the thought of his first date with Ellen. She'd been playing so hard to get. She was always too busy. Finally, he called her up and asked her for Wednesday, Thursday, Friday, Saturday, Sunday, or Monday. She said that Monday might be possible and she'd get back to him. But he could tell she was teasing him. She arrived at his apartment dressed in jeans with a turtleneck. She had her long hair parted down the middle with pigtails. She'd brought a ton of books. It was supposedly a study date. Jack had brought a bottle of Wild Turkey. From the first moment, they played out their roles, she earnestly making rules about studying first and rewarding themselves with a drink later, he putting some bourbon in her Coke and cajoling her into drinking it anyway. They did more fooling around than studying that night.

Jack wondered if she harbored the same fond memories of their first kisses. He smiled and looked back at the journal.

5/1/72. May Day. Ellen's birthday. Sent her a card. "Dear Ellen," I wrote, "I still love you in my fucked-up fashion. Wishing you a Happy Birthday seems like rubbing salt in the wound, so I won't. But do you remember the surprise birthday when I made you keep your eyes closed until we got all the way out to Wingersheek beach and I told you to open them just as a slice of the sun poked out of the sea? We held each other, breathing the salt air, feeling the sun warm our cheeks. Whatever happens. I'll always remember. Whatever happens, I'll always love you, Jack."

"Are you ever coming to bed?" snapped Ellen, as she threw open the door to Jack's office.

Startled, Jack pulled his appointment book over his old journal.

"I'll be there when I'm good and ready," he said without turning around.

"Are you going to keep this up all night?"

"Oh, am I going to keep it up? Who started it?" he said as he wheeled around in his chair.

"Okay, all right then, you win. Satisfied now? I'm too tired to fight. I'm going to bed. Just don't stay up late. I've got to get a decent night's rest."

"Fine, I'll be right up."

"That's what you always say. You don't give a damn about how tired I am." Ellen glowered at him and then stomped off.

Her bathrobe was flapping about her like harpies' wings thought Jack as he watched her retreating back. That woman still has a glare that could burn your skin off. It used to turn his guts to water. Not anymore. Thank Harney for that, he thought.

He began to flip through his journal, looking for his entry about that famous Harney session. He wasn't about to go straight to bed upon Ellen's command.

He felt about 14. He could almost hear Skipper's voice booming up the stairs. "Dinner's on the table. Don't dawdle!"

"Aye, aye, asshole," he'd mutter as he slammed his book shut and hurried to the table.

He found the right page.

7/3/72. Finally. A win for the home team. There I was, slumped down in the chair in my well-practiced adolescent slouch. Ellen was railing at me as usual about what a lying sack of shit I am. I was being nonchalant. I never let her see that she's getting to me. The next thing I knew she was out of the chair and yelling at me, "You're not listening!" and then she kicked me in the shin. I couldn't believe it. Harney leapt out of her chair and went over to Ellen, put her hand on her shoulders, and said, "Ellen, you cannot do that. You can be mad as hell, but you cannot kick Jack." Ellen collapsed back onto the sofa like a rag doll and began crying hard.

I sat straight up. Harney gave me a steady owlish stare and nodded firmly toward Ellen. I looked at Harney and sort of shrugged. Again she gestured toward Ellen, who was holding herself and shaking with sobs.

All of a sudden I could really see Ellen. My heart softened. I got up and knelt next to her. I put my hand gently on the small of her back. "It's okay, I understand. I'm so sorry. I know how much I've hurt you."

Ellen gave me a wild look and then threw her arms around my neck. She started sobbing again. I held her tight.

No matter what. I love her.

Jack sighed and closed the journal. He took off his reading glasses and scratched his bald head. Ellen never really understood how afraid he'd been. Whenever she challenged him, he had simply withdrawn inside his shell, the quintessential turtle. At the time he had no idea how provocative this was for Ellen. The more unreachable he became the more alone and rejected she felt. Naturally she'd keep poking at him and naturally he'd stay tucked up inside himself and try to wait her out. He looked nonchalant, but felt like a little boy.

Ellen's kick and Harney's swift response broke the pattern. Suddenly Ellen wasn't a huge devouring monster about to eat him for breakfast. She wasn't Skipper bellowing at him because he didn't have his shirt tucked in. Ellen had been just as desperate and frightened as he was.

Jack often used this stuff in his therapy with couples, helping women understand better how frightened men can really be and men how provocative and rejecting their withdrawn silence can be. There were a lot of ways that he used the lessons of his and Ellen's marriage more than any teaching he ever received.

The irony was that they would never gone into therapy if it hadn't have been for his stupid affair with Robin. And if they hadn't done the work with Harney, their marriage probably would have imploded later.

They had been so young. Getting married back then seemed a little like playing house. Jack remembered Harney saying that they were like Hansel and Gretel lost in the big dark woods. She used to call his cool posturing his wannabe "James Dean routine," and she told Ellen her scolding tone sounded like the nag in the fairy tale "The Fisherman's Wife." She taught them to laugh at themselves.

What would Harney say if she saw the way they were behaving tonight? They hadn't seen her for a long time. A few years ago Jack heard that her daughter had died. He had planned to write her a note. But he didn't get around to it. He wished he had. She had been such a gift to them. He said out loud, "Screw it, better late than never. I'll write her first thing in the morning."

Jack put the journal away. He was tired. The fight with Ellen seemed terminally stupid. He didn't really know why she'd been so bitchy tonight, anyway. A last-minute therapy cancellation late in the afternoon left him with a big appetite and an unguarded refrigerator. So naturally he wasn't up for her surprise dinner out idea. He was already stuffed. But she'd been very pissy the rest of the night.

But what the hell, he thought, life's short. Maybe a peace offering is in order.

He pulled himself out of his office chair and switched off the light. Perhaps I'll take up a York Peppermint Pattie, he thought, even though it's not exactly a chocolate soufflé.

II

Ellen sat in bed reading *The Lovely Bones*. The book was making her feel worse. This girl watching over her family from heaven after she'd been raped and murdered stirred up her childhood yearnings that someday she'd meet her dad in heaven. She felt part of her was still that 12-year-old girl.

She slammed the book shut. She had been so excited about her plan for the evening. Earlier Megan had called, overflowing with excitement, to tell her that she was going to have a baby, their first grandchild. Ellen almost called Jack immediately but decided to make it into a surprise. She'd made a reservation at Pierre's, their favorite restaurant, and had even pre-ordered the chocolate soufflé dessert for both of them. She called Alex to tell her the news, and she'd been great, none of her little-sister jealousy, even though Alex was dying to get married and have children herself. All the way home in the traffic she had looked forward to the meal and Jack's surprise when she took his hands in hers and said, "Guess what old man? You're going to be a granddad." Maybe they would have shed a few tears together. Maybe they would have made love when they got home.

But, no, he wasn't in the mood to go out. She couldn't change his mind even when she'd told him about the soufflé. So she'd be damned if she'd tell him the good news under those circumstances. After a brief chilly dinner she'd gone off to bed and he had retreated to his lair.

What a dumb night, she thought. Jack looked just like Skipper when he got scowled. Why couldn't he go along with something spontaneous for once? It would have been so nice. He was just staying downstairs on purpose. She decided not to tell him about Megan tonight. She would leave him an "Oh, by the way" note on his desk in the morning.

Ellen gave the pillow a punch and flicked off her nightstand lamp without concern about Jack stumbling in the dark. Serves him right, she thought, as she closed her eyes.

But she was annoyed with herself for being so irritated. After all, it wasn't his fault that he didn't know about the surprise plan. But he was still being a jerk staying up so late—silly sulking man, she smiled. She suddenly could imagine him lying there cradling a little infant in his arms. He would make such a good granddad.

She remembered Jack holding Meggie when she was just a wrinkly tiny bundle in his arms. All she had wanted for the evening was one of those tender moments of holding and being held. She sighed as her anger slipped away. We're way too old for this, she thought, and felt the familiar ache of sadness.

As she curled up, Ellen reached for an old daydream that she hadn't visited in a long while. She had always relied on it when she couldn't sleep as a teenager, and then she did it again during that horrible time when Jack was off on his fling. She would wrap herself in this one moment of memory.

She is seven years old as she jumps off the Oakhill school bus. She's wearing her hair in pigtails and has on her favorite corduroy red jumper and her loafers with bobby socks. After the other kids turn down Hanover Street, she's alone. Alone with her secret companion, her magical mare, Velvet. With a snort and a little buck, they skip down the street toward home. Her hands are bouncing in front of her, lightly holding the reins. Giddy-ap, Giddy-ap—she urges the filly on with a gentle swat on her behind. Her upper body is steady as her legs gallop along. She closes her eyes and feels the powerful surge beneath her, feels the wind blowing through her hair, feels the big Wyoming sky embrace her. Then just as she rounds the corner of her old house, the familiar black Chrysler pulls into the driveway. "Daddy, daddy!" She lets out a shriek of delight and runs to the car. He rolls down the window and puts an arm out to grab her. She leans into the car and kisses him on his scratchy cheek.

"How ya doin', Rootie-patootie," he says with a big smile.

"I'm no Rootie-patootie," she always says with a big smile.

This moment would be forever. She'd be forever riding Velvet home from school and the Chrysler would forever be turning into the driveway.

III

Jack snuck into the bedroom. Ellen was sound asleep. He put the York Peppermint Pattie on her nightstand and undressed quietly.

As he stood over the toilet and waited for his old man trickle to begin, Jack chuckled to himself about the whole stupid evening. It was miracle they had gotten this far. He hoped Megan and Tim could hang in there.

Two nights before Megan's wedding, Ellen had insisted on his having a father–daughter talk with her. "You have no idea how important a dad is to a girl. I'd have given anything if my father had lived to see us get married. You've got to talk with her."

So Jack sat Megan down and plunged in. "Now, I don't need to tell you that marriage is more hard work than giddy romance and more like eating your greens than . . . "

Megan rolled her eyes, "Oh, daddy, I know, trust me." She gave him a big hug and whispered in his ear, "I promise to eat all the brussels sprouts on my plate first."

When he walked Megan down the aisle of St. Andrews, Jack remembered carrying her to the front of the church in her white christening dress 25 years earlier. She was a radiant bride. Once he and Ellen were sitting in the pew together, she had slumped against him and wept. Jack wasn't feeling sad. He felt proud of how far they had come. Hansel and Gretel had found their way through the dark woods after all.

As he slipped into bed next to her, Jack felt a stirring of tenderness. Ellen was curled up with both hands holding the blanket up under her chin. She looked like a little girl. Jack reached over and brushed her hair lightly away from her face. She let out a soft sigh and rolled over. Jack curled up around her spoon fashion. He felt her warmth and the softness of her skin. He put his arm over the swell of her hip. He breathed in the smell of her hair.

QUESTIONS FOR DISCUSSION

1. What do you think of Jack and Ellen's relationship? Would you consider it a successful long-term relationship? Why or why not?
2. Does the kind of conflict and tension that sometimes exist between Jack and Ellen seem typical of most couples?
3. Clearly the work with Dr. Harney helped Jack and Ellen reconcile. Does Jack give her too much credit? How do you feel about the potentially very powerful effect of therapy on the unfolding of people's lives?

4. How is Jack and Ellen's relationship similar to or different from your own experience in relationships?
5. How do you help couples set reasonable expectations for a long-term relationship?
6. Have you been able to set realistic expectations for your relationship? Have they been too high? Too low?

1918

RIDING LESSONS

They called it the spring of memorial services. No burials. The bodies of their boys were over there beneath one of the thousands of white crosses spread across the fields of France. Everyone got used to the sound of Taps and the 21-gun salutes. Since the big German offensive in March, families in Concord had been getting telegrams notifying them of their sons' deaths. The *Boston Globe* reported that Concord had been hit harder then any other town of comparable size in all of New England, and there was even an editorial about the Concord fallen being "Modern Minutemen." First it was the Hinks brothers, Joe and Hank, who had been in the same company; then the Simmons boy, who was all the girls' secret sweetheart; and then Billy Edgerly, who was not well thought of by most folks.

By far the biggest turn out was for Tommy Evans's service. He had been captain of all the high school sports and president of the class of 1911, and everyone thought he would be governor some day. He left behind a young wife and seven-year-old boy.

Tom had been the first in town to volunteer, for the cavalry no less. He was a horseman and they still had cavalry companies back then, although the Army pretty much gave up on horses after the first few months. Most of the town thought he had been very courageous to sign up, even though some whispered that perhaps Concord had become a little small for him, what with living in the same house with his formidable parents and his wife, Millicent, who had always been a little problematic. That marriage had seemed a little suspect to many because of the speedy arrival of little Johnny and because Millicent seemed such an unlikely choice for a man headed for a public life. After all, Millie was a frail wisp who suffered from bouts of female troubles that left her incapacitated for days at a time. She was more than a match for old Doc Blaine, who tried being reassuring and from time to time would give her a tincture of laudanum to take the edge off whatever it was that ailed her.

The day of Captain Evans's memorial service (none of us were surprised that they made him a captain over there, too) was the first truly fine day of May. Concord springs can be cold and wet. This day was bright and clear. There was a soft, warm southerly that kept the flags at half mast rippling a little all through day—"evidence of his presence," Mrs. Goodenough whispered to Mrs. Alcott right in the middle of the service. Everyone commented on what a fine day it was, with folks almost evenly divided about whether good weather made the sad events of the service seem more or less tolerable. Certainly it was an improvement over the snow that came the April morning of the Hinks's service. Everybody froze that day.

Tom Evans's family lived at Shady Hill Farm, which had been purchased in 1872 by General Joshua Evans with the fortune he made from Reconstruction contracts. The morning of the service, Tom's father, Jack, was up before dawn and headed out to the barn. Pop, as everyone called him, had refused to talk to anyone about his son's death. They say that after his wife showed him the telegram, he just clamped his mouth shut and walked away without saying a word. Hadn't said barely a civil word besides "pass the salt" since then. He'd always been a taciturn man, anyway, a true old Yankee: "If you don't have anything good to say then don't say anything at all." One might conclude that over the years, he hadn't had much good to say.

Tom was the sunshine in Pop's life. He basked in the glow of all Tom's accomplishments and promise. Tommy was all Pop really did talk about, and it wasn't just his glory on the athletic fields that he went on about. He liked to talk about Tommy's character and caring for others. Always there for the less fortunate kids. Pop had been sure the boy would make it back. Tom had such a bright future ahead of him.

Pop slid open the barn door and stepped into the gloom. The pungent smell of hay, manure, and horses filled his nostrils. It was like smelling Tommy. Pop's eyes filled with tears. He was surprised by the weakness in his knees, and forced himself to walk down the row of stalls until he came to Tom's horse. Joker was a 25-year-old quarterhorse that Pop had bought when Tommy was seven. Joker and Tommy had been inseparable pals for years.

"Boy spends more time in the barn than he does in the house," complained Tom's mother, Amanda.

Can't say that I blame him, Jack chose not to say out loud.

In the month before he was shipped out, Tom decided the one thing he wanted to do was help his little boy, Johnny, get over his fear of riding. It didn't make sense to Tom. Joker was the easiest horse in the world, but Johnny was still scared. By his son's age Tom had been riding Joker for a year and nobody had ever given him riding lessons. But Johnny needed a little push. It would be good for the boy to take care of Joker while he was gone, Tom thought. Help him grow up a little bit, be a little more manly. The boy had a little too much of his mother in him. Besides, maybe the kid would learn to love to ride. If it worked, he'd buy Johnny a horse when he got back and they could ride together.

Tom carefully walked Johnny through each step of tacking up Joker. He helped him throw the saddle up and pull the cinch tight

As Tom put the bridle on, he said, "I'm counting on you, son. You've got to exercise Joker while I'm gone. You know your mom can't do it and Pop's too old."

"But he's your horse, Daddy. I don't like riding."

"You'll like riding just fine once you get used to it. There's no shame in being a little nervous, boy. But just wait. You'll love being able get out there into the woods and leave everyone behind. Just be on your own. I remember being off for the whole day. Just Joker and me."

Tom paused and patted Joker's neck and said to the horse, "Listen up, I want you to take good care of this kid while I'm gone."

181

The horse flicked his tail at some flies.

Tom turned toward his son. "Now come over here and reach up and grab the pommel and give me your foot." Tom stood there holding the reins with one hand and extending his other toward his son. He was smiling, but his eyes were firm.

Johnny sighed and edged over to where his father was. He tentatively reached up for the pommel. But he couldn't quite reach it.

"Wait a second," said his father. "We've got to get you a stool. You have to be able to do this by yourself."

Tom went and found an old milking stool and positioned it next to the horse. "Go ahead son, get up on that and put your left foot in the stirrup and swing your right up and over."

"Daddy, I can't."

"Of course you can. Don't be afraid."

Johnny shrugged and then he made a lunge at the horse. At the last moment his dad gave him a timely shove on his backside and he made it.

The minute he got astride the horse, Johnny couldn't hold back any longer, and he began to cry.

"Come on, boy, there's nothing to cry about. Let's just give a try, huh?" said Tom as he grabbed the reins to lead the horse toward the paddock.

Johnny nodded, snuffled, and set off slowly. He was able to choke back the tears, but Tom saw how scared and miserable the boy really was and stopped them before horse and rider had completed a lap.

He helped the boy down and said, "Hey, I don't want you worrying too much about this. Not everyone's cut out for horses. When I was a kid, I was afraid of bees. Everybody's afraid of something. You go on back to the house. We'll work on this when you're a little older."

Tom decided to hire the Griffith's son to exercise Joker while he was gone.

The service was going to be at 2 P.M., but Amanda Evans was up early getting the maid, Molly, set up with the silverware polish while she got two pies ready for the oven. There had been offers to help, but Amanda had been firm about wanting to do all the cooking herself. As she busied herself about the kitchen, she decided they might as well have a real breakfast also.

The smells of frying bacon and sausage and the clatter of pots and pans surprised Johnny. Grandma usually didn't do a big country breakfast except on Sundays. Johnny was still in his pajamas. He felt a little guilty about being glad that he didn't have to go to school that day. He was on his hands and knees playing with the lead doughboys his dad had sent home from Paris. He had 12 men in muddy brown uniforms with plate-like helmets. They were carrying rifles on their shoulders with long bayonets, and there was one officer with a sword. That was his dad. Johnny didn't have any other soldiers so his toy farm animals—the horse, the bull, the pig, the cows, and the rest—had to fill in for the Germans.

He'd been playing soldiers a lot since Grandma told him that his dad wasn't coming back, that he'd gone to heaven instead because of being killed. Things didn't seem that different after the news arrived a week ago. His dad had already been gone for a year, so he was kind of used to him not being there. Mother had gone off to bed but that was where she usually was. Grandma was cooking up a storm as always, and Pop was either up in the library or off to the barn by himself. The only thing that seemed much different to Johnny was that all week the kids at school were nicer to him and the grown-ups looked at him with a worried frown as if he were sick or something.

In the battles, the farm animal Germans always appeared to be winning. There were about 25 of them, counting the chickens and the ducks, so they kept overrunning the Yanks' positions. One by one the Yanks would go down until there was only the officer left. He'd draw his sword and charge right at the horse who was the enemy general, but he'd be shot down just like the rest. Then all the Germans would take a nap. But the officer was only pretending to be dead and he'd wake up and stab each German while they were sleeping.

"Johnny," said his mother in a hushed tone.

Johnny looked up from his scene at his sickly-looking mom in her robe.

"You should go down to breakfast now," she whispered and looked straight through him.

"Why are we whispering?" Johnny asked.

She raised her hand and pointed toward her temple. Her arm dropped and she sighed, "I have to rest. We all have to make your father proud today," she muttered as she turned away.

Mother didn't come down for breakfast, so it was just Johnny and Pop and Grandma who served up pancakes, bacon, sausage, and scrambled eggs.

"Jesus, woman, you'd think you were feeding an army, " said Pop as he grabbed for the syrup.

"Don't swear in front of the boy," she snapped back, and then she turned to Johnny, who was sitting in the middle, and smiled. "Have some eggs, Johnny. Fill yourself up. It's going to be a hard day for all of us, even for that cantankerous old man at the end of the table."

Johnny smiled. Nobody messed with Grandma and got away with it. Not even Pop. Johnny was there when the Army man gave her the telegram. She gasped when she read it and put her hand in her mouth and bit hard on it for a second. Then she straightened right up and thanked the man for coming while she tucked the notice in her apron pocket and walked into the kitchen.

"What happened, Grandma?" Johnny asked, as he followed her into the kitchen. She was staring out the window over toward the barn and paddock.

"Your dad's in heaven now, Johnny," she said softly, and then her shoulders began to shake and she started to cry.

Johnny ran to her and gave her a big hug. She gently pushed him away and said, "It's okay. We're going to be okay." He hadn't even been sure what she was talking about, but he was guessing that it meant his daddy had been killed.

They held the service at the family plot out past the north pasture. Reverend Johnson had bowed to the will of Jack Evans, who didn't think much of church in the first place. Pop already had placed a granite marker in the ground. "The service will be a simple a prayer followed by 'Oh God, Our Help in Ages Past.' That's all.

Then there will be a reception back at the house and that will be that," he said to Reverend Johnson in a way that did not welcome alternative ideas.

The whole town was at the service, from the most prominent old families right on down to the shopkeepers and immigrant farmhands. It was more a tribute to Tom than an obligation. Somehow Tom's athletic exploits and his ability to befriend people from all walks of life had made him a true child of the town despite, not because of, the family he came from.

Afterward everyone trooped back to the house, where a huge spread had been laid out on the back veranda. They all knew that Amanda Evans had a reputation for her cooking and would have prepared a splendid feast. So they dug right in while Molly made the rounds with a tray of drinks. For many of them it was their very first time at the Evans house.

There weren't any other kids there and Johnny didn't know what to do with himself. People murmured something at him and patted his head or his shoulder. He wondered how long he'd have to stay there. He wandered over to the big easel where the oil painting of his dad in his Army officer's uniform stood on display. He was looking at his dad and wondering why his dad hadn't gone into the Navy like Uncle Henry, who was safe and sound in a place called Liverpool. He wondered what his dad would think of this big shindig, and where was heaven anyway, and did all this really mean that his dad was never ever coming home?

"Well now, if it isn't the spitting image, " said Mrs. Bronson, patting his head like he was a Lab.

Johnny smiled politely.

"Are you going to be a soldier like your dad when you grow up?" she asked.

Without a moment's thought, Johnny replied, "No, ma'am, I'm going to be a naval officer."

"Trying to be your own little man, are you?" she said in a way that made Johnny's cheeks flush.

"No, ma'am, I mean yes," he stuttered. "Anyway, I have to go, umm, help. Thank you." Johnny fled the room.

In the library, he sat in his grandfather's chair and felt sick. All the bad feelings that he had been successfully keeping at bay swept over him. He felt a tight knot in his stomach. He sat there rubbing his hands up and down his thighs. After a while he began pressing himself in the secret place where the touch of his hand could always comfort him. He suddenly felt flushed with shame and jumped up and went over to his grandfather's desk. There was Pop's prized possession, a handcrafted model of the Wright Brothers' plane that Tom had made when he was a boy and later given to his father as a Christmas present.

Johnny carefully picked up the delicate balsa wood plane and began to fly it around with his hand when the library door opened.

"Boy, what are you doing?" barked his grandfather.

Johnny quickly put the plane down.

"Don't you know how easy to break that thing is?" said Pop, who went over to the desk to make sure it had been put back on the stand properly.

Johnny stuttered some apologies to his grandfather and rushed out the door. He ran straight out of the house. Hot tears streamed down his face. He ran into the barn and flung himself down on a bale of hay and cried hard.

Finally his sobbing subsided and he sat up. His Sunday suit was covered in straw and dust. It had been a long time since he'd been back to the barn. It was dark and musty. When he was littler it gave him the creeps. He noticed that it kind of smelled like his dad. At the end of the row of stalls, Joker was poking his head out and peering at him. He'd been so glad that his dad had gotten Billy Griffiths to take care of Joker. Suddenly, he realized that he hadn't set foot in the barn since that time with his dad trying to get him to ride.

He'd felt so ashamed back then. Why had he been such a scaredy-cat anyway? he wondered. He saw Joker's bridle hanging off the wall and his saddle on a sawhorse right by the stall and he knew what he wanted to do. He was taller now and pretty sure that he could do everything.

Joker pawed the floor when he saw Johnny lift up the saddle. Johnny didn't know why he wasn't frightened. He just wasn't.

"Hey, Joker," he said, as he patted the horse's neck. The horse's ears pricked up and he pawed again. "It's okay, boy."

After Joker was tacked up Johnny looked around for the milking stool, but it was nowhere in sight. He decided he could probably manage on his own.

He led Joker outside by the reins. The paddock was a big dirt ring with an old wood fence. As Joker stood patiently, Johnny reached up and grabbed the pommel with his left hand, lifted his left foot high and jammed it into the stirrup, and flung himself into the saddle. Nothing happened. Joker didn't buck. The saddle didn't fall off. His feet fit in the stirrups.

"Click, click." He made the sound that his dad did and gave Joker a gentle nudge with his heel.

It was getting dark and the reception was thinning out. People were cranking up their Model A Fords, and hitching up their carriages, or untying their horses. There was about an even split between animal and mechanical transportation back then. Everyone sighed and said one more time how sad it was. What a loss for the whole town.

As the slow parade wended down Shady Hill Lane, nobody saw the little boy on the horse. Johnny was alone, galloping Joker around and around the paddock in the gathering twilight.

QUESTIONS FOR DISCUSSION

1. Throughout this book there have been stories about childhood events and their potential impact on adult development. To what degree do you think childhood shapes adult life? How has your life been affected by your childhood?

2. Johnny is quite isolated in his grief. Is this due to the norm of the times, his gender, or both? How might this story have been different if he had been a girl?

3. Tom wants Johnny to become more manly and less fearful by making him take care of his horse. Is this typical fathering behavior? Does it impart masculinity? Is there a particular role that fathers should play in teaching masculinity?

4. Clearly, Tom's death had a dramatic impact on Skipper's life. Given what we have seen of Skipper throughout the book, how would you describe how the loss of a father affected him and also his parenting of Jack? How well do you know your parents' childhood experiences and their impact on how your parents raised you?

EPILOGUE

The bell buoy tolls over the anchorage as the afternoon sea breeze begins to die. My boat, *Crow*, gently rocks to the subsiding swell. Three cormorants wheel in formation by the stern and then inelegantly plop into the water. Overhead the gulls scuffle with each other, fighting for territory with their raucous cries, and there is even the cheep–cheep of an osprey somewhere. Day's end. It's late August and there is a hint of chill in the air despite the cloudless sky and the remaining warmth of the setting sun.

I'm in Damariscove, Maine, a finger of an island that points out to sea near the mouth of Boothbay. Once upon a time, this tiny little harbor was the busiest trading post in the New World. It was easy for the fisherman to get to yet far enough off the coast to make it safe from the hostile locals. Now, 450 years later, it's a wildlife sanctuary for endangered nesting birds as well as the occasional sailor.

I'm on the boat alone, stealing time from family and clients alike to finish this book. Twelve stories are done. It's a small collection. They remind me of the handful of stones my wife always picks up from the hundreds of choices on a rocky Maine beach.

"What makes those stones so special?" I once asked her as we walked back to the boat.

"I don't know. These are just the ones that caught my eye."

189

For 30 years, I have been privileged to be witness to the complex and poignant, miraculous and tragic moments in countless peoples' lives. So many possible stories could have been made up from such rich material. These stories are certainly not a representative sample of all presenting problems. These are just the ones that caught my eye.

These 12 stories are not teaching tales. They don't provide answers, but they pose questions about the nature of therapy and its impact on how peoples' lives unfold. I hope they may provoke you to think about your own clinical work: what you bring to it, how it affects you, what matters the most.

In the preface, I wrote that a friend challenged me not to be satisfied with raising questions but to offer my own reflections on being a therapist after having practiced all these years. This is a daunting task. Yes, I do feel I have accrued some wisdom, but the older I get the more simple and basic it seems to be. Where's the fine line between simple and simplistic?

Last year I went on a retreat with Thich Naht Hanh, the Vietnamese Buddhist teacher. There were 800 of us under a huge tent. It was a middle-aged crowd made up of experienced meditators and practicing Buddhists. As a teacher myself, I was curious how Thict Nat Hanh would engage with such an experienced and knowledgeable audience. After a long wait, this small Vietnamese man swathed in a brown robe, with a shaved head and a lined face, walked slowly across the dais and sat gracefully down on a cushion in front of the microphone. He looked out at the crowd of us, smiled, and nodded. Then he closed his eyes. He sat silently for five full minutes.

Then in a gentle, firm voice, he said, "Sit comfortably. Now, just close your eyes and notice your experience of breathing."

Then he walked the whole group through the very basic teachings of how to meditate. "Just breathe," he said. "Just notice the breath."

Here was one of the most revered spiritual leaders of our times trusting the value of beginning with the beginning.

I'm certainly not Thich Nhat Hanh, but I need to borrow some of his clarity and courage and simply offer a few basic things I've learned about the art and soul of being a therapist from my years of practice. The operative word here is "practice."

GRIEVING ALONE LASTS FOREVER, GRIEVING TOGETHER HEALS

Clients arrive at my office with a huge variety of issues to be worked on: affairs, fights, children, in-laws, addictions, depressions, eating disorders, money, sex, even whose job it is to pick up the socks. Whatever the presenting problems, they usually mask a simple and harsh reality: unresolved grief. At the heart of every therapy is the grief we have about our lives. It may be as dramatic as a childhood violated by neglect and abuse or the death of a loved one, or as simple as getting old and confronting the myriad ways our dreams have faded. It may be our dawning awareness of how truly alone and out of control we are in our lives or our nagging dissatisfaction with our jobs, our relationships, even our children. There is in all of us an abiding yearning for something beyond our reach and a fear of what will ultimately happen to us.

My job in therapy is to help people work on what they can do something about and let go of what they can't. It's as simple as the Serenity Prayer. This inevitably means helping clients give up unrealistic expectations of other people. The people in our lives—parents, partners, friends, and children—can and will sometimes hurt us just by being unreliable, flawed human beings. And despite our best intentions we will also hurt them.

I hate that sometimes I have been harmful to my two sons. Despite loving them unconditionally, I've made mistakes that have hurt them. I tell my clients that the only thing we can truly trust is that love hurts. The challenge in our lives is to risk loving anyway and not shy away or avoid responsibility when we do hurt each other.

It is the same challenge for us therapists. We can never truly be sure if what we do is ultimately helpful or harmful. Therapists are not all-knowing guides marching fearlessly ahead of our clients as we lead them along the harrowing mountain trails. Yes, we do have pitons, ropes, and hammers. We have maps and weather reports, experience and equipment. But these skills don't guarantee our clients' safety or that we will make the summit. Ultimately, our willingness to share the risk, to give gentle voice to the fear, and to hold the sweaty palms is the gift we offer.

Since the beginning of time, humankind has dealt with the inevitable pain of life itself through seeking connection and community. Whether it's a band of Cro-Magnon huddled around a fire underneath the cold canopy of stars or a group of alcoholics in a smoke-filled church basement, the healing words are simply "Me, too." Grieving together heals.

GIVE TIME, TIME

A couple of days ago I heard from Joe, who just wanted me to know that it was his 20th anniversary of sobriety. He was calling to thank me. It's funny. I remember him but I don't remember anything about our therapy. Something happened for him. It was a turning point in his life. I feel humble and bemused. We don't always know the outcome of therapy. We don't necessarily know it 20 years later. We are bit players in the drama of people's lives. Like *Hamlet*'s Rosencrantz and Guildenstern, we arrive in the middle of the play, have our lines, do our turn, but rarely get to see the ending. In the preface I wrote about the follow-up study I did that showed how unpredictable and unreliably reported therapeutic outcomes seem to be. One could be nonplussed. I find it humbling and liberating. Once you learn that sometimes sessions or even whole therapies which seemed to go poorly actually turned out well and that seemingly great sessions can backfire unexpectedly, then you have to learn to let go. Sometimes we have a great impact on people's lives, and sometimes we're just a forgotten name on old check stubs. It takes time for the impact of our work to take root. I remind myself that after the back-breaking effort of planting a new garden, the next morning when one looks out the window, all you'll see is dirt. You have to give it time.

THERAPIST, HEAL THYSELF

For most of us, being a therapist is a calling. Long before graduate school, many of us found our sense of purpose and self-esteem in caring for others. This was the way many of us connected safely.

Relating through care taking is part of what draws many of us to the helping professions. Being a therapist allows us to connect deeply and intimately with people without having to be equally exposed and vulnerable. It creates potentially a kind of ersatz intimacy, in which the therapist is fully emotionally present, but on his terms and within the boundaries of the professional relationship. Personally, being a wise and loving clinician has been a lot easier for me than being a husband, father, or friend. For years my emotional needs were too often more easily met in the safety of my role as a therapist. Empathically connecting and helping with my clients' pain allowed me to vicariously work on my own unresolved grief from the relative immunity of the therapist's chair. Like some of the therapists portrayed in the stories, I too have often given my clients my best self, while giving my family only leftovers.

All of us have a profound responsibility to make sure our work, our caring, our love is in the service of our clients and not ourselves. Our vulnerability allows us to deeply connect to our clients, but it can impair our judgment and potentially cause harm. It's essential that we fully and repeatedly explore and work on our own emotional issues throughout our professional lives.

It is also critically important that none of us practice without ongoing support and supervision. We do not practice a knowable science. We are practitioners of a mysterious art. There are so many ways to make mistakes, overlook something, and get stuck that we all need to be reviewing our cases with a peer group or supervisor to matter how senior we may be.

There have been times in my career when out of my own mix of hubris and embarrassment I have not followed this sage advice. Pride has led me to make mistakes and harm some of my clients. We teach our clients to ask for help scaling the difficult mountains in their lives, yet sometimes we think we should be able to do the climb alone. That's not safe for you or your clients.

GRACE HAPPENS

Part of being a healer is to have our own centering practice in which we connect our small, insignificant lives to a pattern of meaning in the universe in whatever way we understand it. This sense of perspective allows us to stay humble as we respond to our clients' suffering and risk having a powerful impact on their lives.

Many of us struggle to reconcile our rational minds and our yearning for spiritual connection. Years ago, a friend of mine presented a lowest common denominator description of the Higher Power that bypasses tangled questions of God and gets to the heart of the matter. We were presenting on the subject of spirituality and AA. My friend, a talented social worker and a longtime member of AA, has a tough, blunt speaking style that sometimes is belied by the twinkle in her eye.

She said to her audience, "When I was an active drunk, I was an atheist and I didn't believe in any of this God crap! Now I've been sober for 15 years and I still don't believe in any of this God crap!"

The startled audience froze. She glared at them and went on. "There's only one thing you need to know to have the healing presence of the Higher Power in your life."

She paused. You could have heard a pin drop. "The only thing you need to know about the Higher Power is You're Not It!"

Time and again I've walked into my office about to see dangerous, suicidal, out-of-control clients and repeated to myself the mantra "Remember, David, you're not it." Then I ask for help. I don't know if God is on the other end of the line when I pray, but I do know that prayer is good for me. It puts me in right relationship to the universe.

It puts me in touch with how little I am. It breaks through my grandiose self-importance and sense of responsibility. It's not all about me.

My job is to do my best. But our best efforts don't ensure that the therapy will help or even that we won't do harm. I have on my desk a Jew's harp. Elena, a client whom I'd treated after her husband had had an affair, gave it to me. She went through a tumultuous divorce and a profound grief response. We worked well together. She gave the present to me as a part of our ending. Nine months after our last session, she came in for what she referred to as a tune-up. She seemed to be in good shape. I was quite complimentary about the progress that she had made, and it felt like an affirming session. Two weeks later, Elena killed herself. There must have been some clues, but I didn't see them.

I keep the Jew's harp in front of me so that I might never forget her and to stay fully alert to the people sitting in front of me. I will never know if there was something I might have said or done that could have made a difference. This is the risk we take every day.

After all the theories are considered and the techniques are applied, the best we have to offer our clients is our own flawed humanity as we care for them as well as we can. If we do our best, then Grace happens. Sometimes.

HAVE FUN

Part of being a therapist is accepting that you will always make mistakes, that the more you learn the more you'll realize how much you don't know. Our obligation to all who come to us is to learn from our mistakes, recognize our limitations, and resist taking ourselves too seriously. We need to be able to experience the joy of tears and the tears of joy.

Thirty years ago, when I was filled with grandiose seriousness about being a therapist, my first supervisor, Robert Klein, put his arm on my shoulder, looked at me with a twinkle his eye, and said, "Remember, David, it's got to be fun."

At the time I was affronted by what seemed like such a facetious remark. But after a lifetime of sitting with the tragedies and foibles of my clients' lives, it turns out he was right. You have to truly enjoy the majesty and mystery of engaging people and becoming a part of their lives for a time. It has to be fun.

*   *   *

The throaty rumble of the lobster boat and the toss of its wake combine to wake me up. It's still dark, but my watch says it's 7:15. I get out of my warm bag and poke my nose up through the hatch. The fog has rolled in. I'm in this tiny harbor and can barely make out the ghostly outlines of the shore. "It's thick o' fog" as they say Down East.

Today is my last writing day. I've got to get home. It won't be so hard leaving this place in this stuff, but I hope it lifts before I get to my home port, which can be a little tricky to sail into in the fog.

I'm afraid that what I wrote last night doesn't convey the richness of therapy, the privileges and responsibilities of being a therapist, and the serendipitous surprises of life itself. I remember one of my AA clients leaning forward as if to take me into his confidence and saying in his gravelly smoker's voice, "You know, Doc, you don't know what you don't know!"

He was right. That's why I wrote these stories. It seemed a better way of exploring how much we don't know. Some of the time we do have to sail through the fog. With careful practice, we can learn to do it well. And slowly as the sun burns through the clouds, the fog lifts and we can see clearly.

STUDY GUIDE

I wrote these stories for all of us—novice and veteran—in the care giving professions. The challenges of being a therapist constantly change, yet never are fully resolved, even in a lifetime of practice. These stories are a different way of looking at and discussing those challenges. Each of them evokes themes related to the issues people bring to therapy, the impact of therapy on the client and therapist, the personal life and private thoughts of the therapist, and the unpredictability of our lives over time.

I wrote these stories with four different readers in mind: graduate students in clinical training programs, peer supervision groups, book groups, and individual clinicians. At the end of each story is a series of questions intended to stimulate readers to explore the relevance of the story to their own work and personal life.

FOR GRADUATE STUDENTS

Because these stories explore the lives of clients and therapists alike, they can break down the distance that often separates the new clinician from the experience of his or her clients. The stories also allow students to explore their projections about what a therapist is supposed to be like in both their personal and professional lives. Students need to learn that therapists are just human beings struggling alongside their clients. Thus a story like "Malibu Barbie Loves You" is important because a student can see that one can be struggling in one's personal life and still be a gifted and successful clinician. Many of the stories allow the new clinician to explore questions about the profession, its rewards, and its personal cost in a way quite different from standard textbooks and manuals. Most good textbooks have at least a chapter on the importance of therapeutic boundaries and professional ethics, but I hope "Heart to Heart" shows the potential dangers of transgression resulting from the intense intimacy of psychotherapy and a therapist's emotional vulnerability. The stories will provoke heated discussion and personal insights, which may lead to much greater self-awareness and appreciation for how truly challenging the practice of psychotherapy can be.

The book can serve as a challenging, yet appealing, primary text in a graduate course about the nature of therapy and of being a therapist. The book could also be utilized as a supplementary text, helping students explore general clinical issues in a much more personal way.

In a semester-long seminar, the leader can assign students one story for each class, followed by in-class discussion of the answers to the questions. The questions at the end of each story explore three areas: clinical issues, the nature of therapy, and the readers' relevant personal experiences. The in-class discussion would focus first on the clinical issues being addressed and then move to encouraging the students to think in new ways about their personal lives and their lives as therapists. Some stories may evoke concerns about being a therapist that wouldn't otherwise surface. Or they may raise personal issues. Stories like "The Morning of February Fifth" can be very fruitful, even if difficult, for students who are survivors of a family member's suicide. Such classes can lead to powerful group discussions about how to handle vulnerabilities and fears as a student and as a therapist. The teacher and seminar leader might offer students private time to discuss issues they didn't want to address in the group.

Students would be encouraged to read and discuss just one story at a time because many of the stories have surprising sequels. For example, the couple in "Lunar Missions" has a tender reconciliation; years later, in "Dress-Ups," we discover that the transgender issues actually led to the breakup of the marriage. Following these characters and relationships over time will allow students to reexamine their responses as events unfold. Students will also be able to examine their assumptions about how life unfolds and how we understand the relationships between events at one stage of life and events that happen at other stages.

To use the stories as supplemental course reading, teachers can assign their students particular stories or the entire book and ask them to write a paper on a variety of topics. For instance, the assignment might be to read "Bleeding the Lines" and write a paper about grief and healing or to read "Not Exactly a Chocolate Soufflé" and discuss the students' assumptions and experiences with long-term relationships.

PEER SUPERVISION GROUPS

Practicing clinicians know better than anyone the constant challenge to stay fresh and renewed with their clients. This collection of stories supplies peer supervision groups a way to explore collectively the troubling dilemmas we all face in the course of doing psychotherapy. Each member of the peer group might use one particular story or a recurring theme that had meaning to them and lead a discussion about those issues and how they apply in their own clinical practice and personal lives. Or the group members might use the stories to discuss current problems they are having with a particular case, client, or personal issue. For instance, a therapist at an impasse with a suicidal and severely traumatized client might find it useful to discuss the difficulties that Jack Evans was experiencing in his work with Ann in "Split Rock Gorge." Clearly, it was a case that he was struggling with and that he needed to override his pride to get help on. Sometimes in my supervision groups, therapists have a hard time talking about their most difficult cases because they are too embarrassed by their feelings of inadequacy. Yet all of us have experienced cases in which we've made mistakes, and even done harm. Discussing the issues in the story may make it safer for clinicians to share their own struggles.

BOOK GROUPS

Book groups comprising both clinicians and lay people might use this book as a springboard to discuss the nature of therapy itself, the variety of ways people confront or avoid problems, and the unexpected changes that turn our lives around. A group of nontherapists can use this book as an entry point to explore their attitudes about therapy, its potentially positive and/or harmful effects, and the role it plays in their own or their friends' lives. Book groups can also explore the efficacy of using fiction rather than case studies, or the effect on the stories and book as a whole of having recurring characters and situations.

For Individual Readers

I encourage individuals to read this book with a friend or family member. Discuss it, argue about it, pick it apart, consider how it applies to your lives. Having participated in a book group myself, and having read and discussed many books with my wife, I'm convinced that sharing and comparing the impact and feelings that a book engenders is critical to fully appreciating it, and to taking all it has to offer. So, if you want to fully explore this book to know yourself and others better, share it and your thoughts with a friend.

And, above all, enjoy.

SUGGESTED READINGS

LUNAR MISSIONS

(impact of family of origin on a couple's intimacy and sexuality; cross-dressing; couple therapy)

Boyd, H. (2004). *My Husband Betty: Love, Sex and Life with a Cross-Dresser.* New York: Thunder's Mouth Press.

Brown, G. R. (1995). "Transvestitism," in *Treatments of Psychiatric Disorders*, G. O. Gabbard, ed. Washington, DC: American Psychiatric Press.

Carnes, P. (2001). *Out of the Shadows: Understanding Sexual Addiction.* Center City, MN: Hazelden Information Center.

Carnes, P. (1997). *The Betrayal Bond.* Deerfield Beach, FL: Health Communications.

Christensen, A., & Jacobson, N. (1999). *Reconcilable Differences.* New York: Guilford Press.

Dattilio, F. M. (2001). *Case Studies in Couple and Family Therapy: Systemic and Cognitive Perspectives.* New York: Guilford Press.

Hendrix, H. (1997). *Giving the Love That Heals.* New York: Simon & Schuster.

Hendrix, H. (1992). *Getting the Love You Want: A Guide for Couples.* New York: Henry Holt.

Jacobson, N., & Christensen, A. (1998). *Acceptance and Change in Couples Therapy: A Therapist's Guide to Transforming Relationships.* New York: Norton.

Leiblum, S., & Rosen, R. C. (2000). *Principles and Practices of Sex Therapy.* New York: Guilford Press.

McCarthy, B. (2004). *Rekindling Desire: A Step-by-Step Program to Help Low-Sex and No-Sex Marriages.* New York: Brunner-Routledge.

Mellody, P., & Freundlich, L. S. (2003). *The Intimacy Factor: The Ground Rules for Overcoming the Obstacles to Truth, Respect, and Lasting Love.* San Francisco: HarperCollins.

Papp, P. (ed.). (2001). *Couples on the Fault Line: New Directions for Therapists.* New York: Guilford Press.

Perel, E. (2003, May/June). "Erotic Intelligence: Reconciling Sensuality and Domesticity," *Psychotherapy Networker*, 25ff.

Schnarch, D. A. (1991). *Constructing the Sexual Crucible: An Integration of Sexual and Marital Therapy.* New York: Norton.

Walker, M., & Rosen, W. (2004). *How Connections Heal: Stories from Relational-Cultural Therapy.* New York: Guilford Press.

MALIBU BARBIE LOVES YOU

(extramarital relationships; person of the therapist; couple therapy; parenting)

DiBlasio, F. A. (2000). "Forgiveness Therapy in Cases of Marital Infidelity," *Psychotherapy, 37*(2), 149–158.

Efran, J. (2002, March/April). "To Tell the Truth: Letting Go of Our Inscrutable Façade," *Psychotherapy Networker*, 35ff.

Enright, R.D. (2001). *Forgiveness Is a Choice: A Step-by-Step Process for Resolving Anger and Restoring Hope.* Washington, DC: American Psychological Association Press.

Enright, R., & North, J. (1998). *Exploring Forgiveness.* Madison: University of Wisconsin Press.

Geller, J. D., Norcross, J., & Orlinsky, D. (2004). *The Psychotherapist's Own Psychotherapy: Patient and Client Perspectives.* New York: Oxford University Press.

Genova, P. (2000). *The Thaw: 24 Essays in Psychotherapy.* Pittsburgh: Dorrance.

Jauregui, A. (2003). *Epiphanies: A Psychotherapist's Tales of Spontaneous Emotional Healing.* New York: Prima.

Layton, M. (1998, November/December). "Ripped Apart: What Does It Take to Turn Bitter Obsession into Forgiveness?" *Family Therapy Networker* [now *Psychotherapy Networker*], 24–31.

Spring, J. (1996). *After the Affair: Healing the Pain and Rebuilding Trust When a Partner Has Been Unfaithful.* New York: HarperCollins.

MAJOR GOATS

(adolescent substance abuse; family therapy; adolescent peer relationships)

Diamond, J. (2002). *Narrative Means to Sober Ends: Treating Addiction and Its Aftermath.* New York: Guilford Press.

Hanna, F. J., & Hunt, W. P. (1999). "Techniques for Psychotherapy with Defiant, Aggressive Adolescents," *Psychotherapy, 36*(1), 56–68.

Liddle, H. A., et al. (2002). "Multidimensional Family Therapy for Adolescent Drug Abuse: Results of a Randomized Clinical Trial," *American Journal of Drug and Alcohol Abuse, 27*(4), 651–688.

Monti, P. M, Colby, S. M., & O'Leary, T. A. (eds.). (2001). *Adolescents, Alcohol, and Substance Abuse: Reaching Teens through Brief Interventions.* New York: Guilford Press.

Selekman, M. (2003). *Solution-Focused Therapy with Children: Harnessing Family Strengths for Systemic Change*. New York: Guilford Press.

Selekman, M. (2002). *Living on the Razor's Edge: Solution-Oriented Brief Family Therapy with Self-Harming Adolescents*. New York: Norton.

Taffel, R. (2000). *Getting through to Difficult Kids and Parents: Uncommon Sense for Child Professionals*. New York: Guilford Press.

Treadway, D. C. (1989). *Before It's Too Late: Working with Substance Abuse in the Family*. New York: Norton.

SPLIT ROCK GORGE

(trauma survivors; transference and countertransference;
sexual abuse; boundaries in the therapeutic relationship)

Chu, J. (1988). "Ten Traps for Therapists in the Treatment of Trauma Survivors," *Dissociation, 1*, 24–32.

Chu, J. (1998). *Rebuilding Shattered Lives: The Responsible Treatment of Complex Post-Traumatic and Dissociative Disorders*. Hoboken, NJ: Wiley.

Dalenberg, C. (2000). *Countertransference and the Treatment of Trauma*. Washington, DC: American Psychological Association Press.

Davies, J. M., & Frawley, M. G. (1994). *Treating the Adult Survivor of Childhood Sexual Abuse*. Boulder, CO: Perseus Books.

Herman, J. (1997). *Trauma and Recovery: The Aftermath of Violence-From Domestic Abuse to Political Terror*. Boulder, CO: Basic Books.

Linehan, M. (1993). *Cognitive-Behavioral Treatment of Borderline Personality Disorder*. New York: Guilford Press.

Linehan, M. (2003). *From Suffering to Freedom: Practicing Reality Acceptance* [videotape]. New York: Guilford Press.

Norcross, J. C., & Goldfried, M. R. (eds.). (2003). *Handbook of Psychotherapy Integration*. New York: Oxford University Press.

DRESS-UPS

(grief; child's loss of a parent; forgiveness; transgender)

Dowrick, S. (1997). *Forgiveness and Other Acts of Love: Courage, Restraint, Forgiveness, Generosity, Tolerance, Fidelity*. New York: Norton.

Eagly, A. H., Beall, A. E., & Sternberg, R. J. (eds.). (2004). *The Psychology of Gender* (2nd ed.). New York: Guilford Press.

Ettner, R. (1999). *Gender Loving Care: A Guide to Counseling Gender-Variant Clients*. New York: Norton.

Lev, A. I. (2003). *Transgender Emergence: Counseling Gender-Variant People and Their Families*. Binghamton, NY: Haworth Press.

Neimeyer, R. A. (2001). *Meaning Reconstruction and the Experience of Loss*. Washington, DC: American Psychological Association Press

Neimeyer, R. A. (1998). *Lessons of Loss: A Guide to Coping*. New York: McGraw-Hill.

Simon, R., Markowitz, L., Barrilleaux, C., & Topping, B. (eds.). (1999). *The Art of Psychotherapy: Case Studies from the Family Therapy Networker*. New York: Jossey-Bass.

Walsh, F., & McGoldrick, M. (2004). *Living Beyond Loss: Death in the Family* (2nd ed.). New York: Norton.

HEART TO HEART

(therapeutic boundary issues; ethical and legal
dilemmas; erotic transference)

Barrett. M. J. (2002, March/April). "The Crush: Challenging our Culture of Avoidance," *Psychotherapy Networker*, 41ff.

Bates, C. M., & Brodsky, A. M. (1993). *Sex in the Therapy Hour: A Case of Professional Incest*. New York: Guilford Press.

Lazarus, A. (2003, March/April). "A Triple Boundary Crossing: From Client to Friend to Client," *Psychotherapy Networker*, 47ff.

Pope, K. S. (2000). "Therapists' Sexual Feelings and Behaviors," in *Psychological Perspectives on Human Sexuality*, L. Szuchman & F. Muscarella, eds. Hoboken, NJ: Wiley.

Pope, K. S., & Vasquez, M. J. T. (1998). "Dual Relationships Scenarios and Questions," from the chapter "Multiple Relationships," in *Ethics in Psychotherapy and Counseling: A Practical Guide* (2nd ed.). San Francisco: Jossey-Bass.

Reamer, F. G. (1999). *Social Work Values and Ethics* (2nd ed.). New York: Columbia University Press.

Rowen, S. (2002, March/April). "The Slippery Slope: Violating the Ultimate Therapeutic Taboo," *Psychotherapy Networker*, 38ff.

Schamess, G. (1999). "Therapeutic Love and Its Permutations," *Clinical Social Work Journal, 27*(1), 9–26.

Simon, R. I. (1995). "The Natural History of Therapist Sexual Misconduct: Identification and Prevention," *Psychiatric Annals, 24,* 509–515.

Simon, R. I. (1999). "Therapist–Patient Sex: From Boundary Violations to Sexual Misconduct," *Psychiatric Clinics of North America, 22,* 31–47.

Younggren, J. N. (2002). "Ethical Decision-Making and Dual Relationships," available online at: *www.kspope.com*

Zur, O. (2004). "Guidelines for Non-Sexual Dual Relations and Boundaries in Psychotherapy," available online at: *www.drozur.com/dualrelationships. Html*

BLEEDING THE LINES

(grief; impact of a child's death on parents; therapist's own recovery)

Becvar, D. S. (2003). *In the Presence of Grief: Helping Family Members Resolve Death, Dying, and Bereavement Issues*. New York: Guilford Press.

Boerner, K., & Heckhausen, J. (2003). "To Have and Have Not: Adaptive Bereavement by Transforming Mental Ties to the Deceased," *Death Studies, 27*(3), 199–226.

Greenspan, M. (2003). *Healing through Dark Emotions: The Wisdom of Grief, Fear and Despair.* Boston: Shambhala.

Kubler-Ross, E. (1997). *On Death and Dying: What the Dying Have to Teach Doctors, Nurses, Clergy and Their Own Families.* New York: Scribner.

Murphy, S., Johnson, L. C., & Lohan, J. (2002). "The Aftermath of the Violent Death of a Child: An Integration of the Assessments of Parents' Mental Distress and PTSD during the First Five Years of Bereavement," *Journal of Loss and Trauma, 7*, 203–222.

Murphy, S., Johnson, L. C., Lohan, J., & Tapper, V. J. (2002). "Bereaved Parents' Use of Individual, Family and Community Resources 4 to 60 Months after a Child's Violent Death," *Family Community Health, 25*(1), 75–82.

Stroebe, M., van Son, M., Stroebe, W., et al. (2000). "On the Classification and Diagnosis of Pathological Grief," *Clinical Psychological Review, 20*(1), 57–75.

Wogrin, C. (2001). *Matters of Life and Death: Finding the Words to Say Goodbye.* New York: Random House.

Wortman, C., & Silver, R. (2001). "The Myths of Coping with Loss Revisited," in *Handbook of Bereavement Research: Consequences, Coping and Care*, M. Stroebe et al., eds. Washington, DC: American Psychological Association Press

THE MORNING OF FEBRUARY FIFTH

(suicidality; depression; impact of suicide on families)

Dunne, E., McIntosh, J., & Dunne-Maxim, K (1987). *Suicide and Its Aftermath: Understanding and Counseling the Survivors.* New York: Norton.

McCracken, A., & Semel, M. (1999). *A Broken Heart Still Beats.* Center City, MN: Hazelden.

Mishara, B. L. (ed.). (1995). *The Impact of Suicide.* New York: Springer.

Moody, R. (2002). *The Black Veil: A Memoir with Digressions.* New York: Little Brown.

Shneidman, E. (2001). *Comprehending Suicide: Landmarks in 20th Century Suicidology.* Washington, DC: American Psychological Association Press.

Solomon, A. (2002). *The Noonday Demon: An Atlas of Depression.* New York: Scribner.

Stimming, M. T., & Stimming, M. (eds.). (1999). *Before Their Time: Adult Children's Experiences of Parental Suicide.* Philadelphia: Temple University Press.

Styron, W. (1990). *Darkness Visible: A Memoir of Madness.* New York: Random House.

Treadway, D. (1996). *Dead Reckoning: A Therapist Confronts His Own Grief.* Boulder, CO: Basic Books.

THE AMERICAN CAB COMPANY

(burnout and therapist self-care; the community of clinicians;
the power of sharing grief)

Akeret, R. A. (1995). *Tales from a Traveling Couch: A Psychotherapist Revisits His Most Memorable Patients*. New York: Norton.

Baker, E. K. (2003). *Caring for Ourselves: A Therapist's Guide to Personal and Professional Well-Being*. Washington, DC: American Psychological Association Press.

Figley, C. R. (2002). "Compassion Fatigue: Psychotherapists' Chronic Lack of Self Care," *Journal of Clinical Psychology, 58*(11), 1433–1441.

Fraenkel, P. (2001, November/December). "The New Normal: Living with a Transformed Reality," *Psychotherapy Networker,* 20ff.

Goldfein, J. S. (2004, January/February). "Reclaiming the Self: One Woman's Refusal to Allow a Nightmare to Define Her Life," *Psychotherapy Networker,* 47–55.

Grosch, W., & Olsen, D. C. (1994). *When Helping Starts to Hurt*. New York: Norton.

Moore, T. (2003). *Care of the Soul: A Guide for Cultivating Depth and Sacredness in Everyday Life*. New York: HarperCollins.

Oliver, M. (1993). *New and Selected Poems*. Boston: Beacon Press.

Skovholt, T. (2001). *The Resilient Practitioner: Burnout Prevention and Self-Care Strategies for Counselors, Therapists, Teachers and Health Care Professionals*. Boston: Allyn & Bacon.

Sussman, M. B. (ed.). (1995). *A Perilous Calling: The Hazards of Psychotherapy Practice*. New York: Wiley.

Treadway, D. (1998, January/February). "Riding Out the Storm," *Family Therapy Networker* [now *Psychotherapy Networker*], 54–61.

White, M. (1997). *Narratives of Therapists' Lives*. Adelaide, Australia: Dulwich Centre Publications.

INTO THE WILD BLUE

(three-generation family dynamics; therapists' own families;
family communications; war trauma)

Davis, J. M., et al. (1996). "Physiological Arousal and Attention in Veterans with Post-Traumatic Stress Disorder," *Journal of Psychopathology and Behavioral Assessment, 18*(1), 1–20.

Dickey, C. (1999). *Summer of Deliverance: A Memoir of Father and Son*. New York: Touchstone Books.

Durst, N. (2003). "Child Survivors of the Holocaust: Age-Specific Traumatization and the Consequences for Therapy," *American Journal of Psychotherapy, 57*(4), 499–518.

Fleming, W. (2003, September/October). "War Stories: When Children Live Out Their Fathers' Traumas," *Psychotherapy Networker,* 96.

Foisson, P., Rejas, M., Pelk, I., & Hirsch, S. (2003). "Family Approach with Grandchildren of Holocaust Survivors," *American Journal of Psychotherapy, 57*(4), 519–527.

Gilroy, P., Carroll, L., & Murra, J. (2002). "A Preliminary Survey of Psychologists' Personal Experiences with Depression and Treatment," *Professional Psychology: Research and Practice, 33*, 402–407.

Kaup, B. A., Ruskin, P. E., & Nyman, G. W. (1994). "Significant Life Events and PTSD in Elderly World War II Veterans," *American Journal of Geriatric Psychiatry, 2*(3), 239–243.

Walsh, F. (2002). *Normal Family Processes: Growing, Diversity, and Complexity* (3rd ed.) New York: Guilford Press.

Van der Kolk, B., McFarlane, A. C., & Weisaeth, L. (eds.). (1996). *Traumatic Stress: The Effects of Overwhelming Experience on Mind, Body, and Society*. New York: Guilford Press.

NOT EXACTLY A CHOCOLATE SOUFFLÉ

*(long-term couple relationships; developmental stages
of couple relationships; therapist's self care)*

Cooper, G. (2003, March/April). "Befriending the Giant," *Psychotherapy Networker,* 34ff.

Dym, B., & Glenn, M. L. (1993). *Couples: Exploring and Understanding the Cycles of Intimate Relationships*. San Francisco: HarperCollins.

Gilligan, S. (2001, January/February). "Getting to the Core: Mastering the Art of Therapeutic Connection," *Family Therapy Networker* [now *Psychotherapy Networker*], 22ff.

Gottman, J. M. (1999). *The Marriage Clinic: A Scientifically Based Marital Therapy*. New York: Norton.

Johnson, S. M. (1996). *The Practice of Emotionally Focused Marital Therapy: Creating Connection*. New York: Taylor & Francis.

Johnson, S. M., & Whiffen, V. E. (eds.). (2003). *Attachment Processes in Couple and Family Therapy*. New York: Guilford Press.

Viorst, J. (2003). *Grown-Up Marriage: What We Know, Wish We Had Known, and Still Need to Know About Being Married*. New York: Simon & Schuster.

Welwood, J. (1996). *Love and Awakening: Discovering the Sacred Path of Intimate Relationship*. New York: HarperCollins.

RIDING LESSONS

*(fathers and sons; masculinity and grief;
childhood loss and its lifelong impact)*

Bohart, A., & Tallman, K. (1999). *How Clients Make Therapy Work: The Process of Active Self-Healing*. Washington, DC: American Psychological Association Press.

Daniel, J. L., & Daniel, O. C. (2003). *We Fish: The Journey to Fatherhood.* Pittsburgh, PA: University of Pittsburgh Press.

Duncan, B. L., Miller, S. D., & Sparks, J. A. (2004). *The Heroic Client.* New York: Wiley.

Lambert, M. J. (2003). *Bergin and Garfield's Handbook of Psychotherapy and Behavior Change* (5th ed.). New York: Wiley.

Lieblich, A., McAdams, D. P., & Josselson, R. (2004). *Healing Plots: The Narrative Basis of Psychotherapy.* Washington, DC: American Psychological Association Press.

Real, T. (1998). *I Don't Want to Talk About It: Overcoming the Secret Legacy of Male Depression.* New York: Simon & Schuster.

Woolfolk, R. L. (1998). *The Cure of Souls: Science, Values and Psychotherapy.* San Francisco: Jossey-Bass.

Worden, J. W. (2002). *Children and Grief: When a Parent Dies.* New York: Guilford Press.

EPILOGUE

*(the practice of psychotherapy; spirituality;
integration of therapist's personal and professional life)*

Brach, T. (2004). *Radical Acceptance: Embracing Your Life with the Heart of a Buddha.* New York: Bantam.

Elridge, N., Surrey, J., Rosen, W., & Baker Miller, J. (2003). *What Changes in Therapy? Who Changes?* Wellesley, MA: Stone Center.

Framo, J. L., Weber, T., & Levine, F. (2003). *Coming Home Again: A Family-of-Origin Consultation.* New York: Brunner-Routledge.

Gilligan, S. (1997). *The Courage to Love: Principles and Practices of Self-Relations Psychotherapy.* New York: Norton.

Gilligan, S. (2003, January/February). "Getting to the Core," *Psychotherapy Networker,* 22ff.

Goleman, D. (2003). *Destructive Emotions: How Can We Overcome Them? A Scientific Collaboration with the Dalai Lama.* New York: Bantam Books.

Siegel, S. (1999). *The Patient Who Cured His Therapist, and Other Stories of Unconventional Therapy.* New York: Marlowe.

Simon, G. (2002). *Beyond Technique in Family Therapy: Finding Your Therapeutic Voice.* Boston: Allyn & Bacon.

Stern, D. (2004). *The Present Moment in Psychotherapy and Everyday Life.* New York: Norton.

Yalom, I. D. (1990). *Love's Executioner, and Other Tales of Psychotherapy.* San Francisco: HarperCollins.

Yalom, I. D. (1992). *When Nietzsche Wept.* Hoboken, NJ: Basic Books.